Praise for *Pick Your Yoga Practice*

"Until Meagan McCrary's book, choosing the right style of yoga was like blind dating. You'd have to try various styles before finding the one for you. Now, finally, there's a guidebook. Let this book be your yoga matchmaker."

— Brian Leaf, author of *Misadventures of a Garden State Yogi*

"Meagan McCrary's book is perfect not only for those who are wondering how to choose a yoga class or style but also for those who are interested in an intelligent and thorough historical account of these yoga styles and their evolution in the West. This is a much-needed asset for anyone who's ever been overwhelmed by the diversity of yoga methods out there!"

— Amy Ippoliti, yoga teacher and cofounder of 90 Monkeys

PICK YOUR
YOGA
PRACTICE

PICK YOUR YOGA PRACTICE

EXPLORING AND UNDERSTANDING
DIFFERENT STYLES OF YOGA

MEAGAN McCRARY

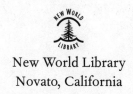

New World Library
Novato, California

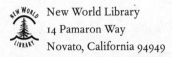

New World Library
14 Pamaron Way
Novato, California 94949

The material in this book is intended for education. Please consult a qualified health care practitioner before beginning any exercise program.

Text design by Tona Pearce Myers

Library of Congress Cataloging-in-Publication Data
McCrary, Meagan, author.
 Pick your yoga practice : exploring and understanding different styles of yoga / Meagan McCrary.
   pages   cm
Includes bibliographical references and index.
ISBN 978-1-60868-180-8 (pbk.) — ISBN 978-1-60868-181-5 (ebook)
1. Hatha yoga. 2. Yoga. 3. Exercise. I. Title.
RA781.7.M399 2013
613.7'046—dc23   2013032437

First printing, December 2013
ISBN 978-1-60868-180-8
Printed in Canada on 100% postconsumer-waste recycled paper

 New World Library is proud to be a Gold Certified Environmentally Responsible Publisher. Publisher certification awarded by Green Press Initiative. www.greenpressinitiative.org

10 9 8 7 6 5 4 3 2 1

Pick Your Yoga Practice is dedicated to my grandma.
Without her, this book would never have been possible.
She has blessed my life beyond measure —
there are no words for the depth of my gratitude.
I love you, my fairy godmother.

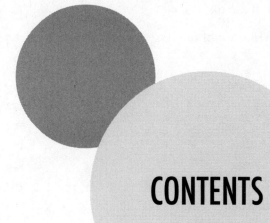

CONTENTS

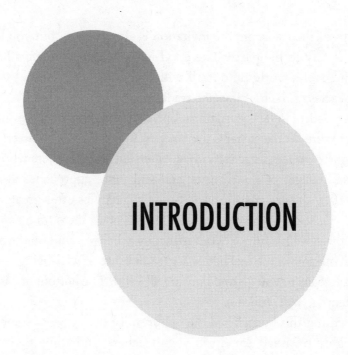

INTRODUCTION

Before I dive into describing the individual styles of yoga, you should know that there are more commonalities to the yoga practices than there are differences. In the end, they all offer you the opportunity to become quiet and just be with yourself, a way of exploring and getting to know yourself, and a technique for moving and breathing in your body, and they all promote mindfulness and presence and seek to expand self-awareness. The goal is the same: to grow as conscious beings. Professor Douglas Brooks, a Hindu scholar, once defined yoga as the "virtuosity in becoming yourself" — a continual refinement of your own authentic expression. The more esoteric definition or goal of yoga is to achieve union with the Divine, God, supreme consciousness, the universe, or whatever you want to call it.

The thing about yoga is this: There's so much more than what appears on the surface. Layered like an onion, the tradition is rich in concepts and ideas, philosophies and mythoi, rituals and practices, and so forth. However, for the most part, yoga is not going to overtly present the deeper meanings of the tradition; the invitation is always open, but you have to find your way to the party. The good news is, once you start looking, you'll discover a world unto itself with plenty of opportunities to study the intricacies of the multifaceted tradition.

A myriad of styles, variations, and combinations of yoga practices exist out there. Some systems are steeped in tradition with direct ties to Indian gurus, others were started by American yoga teachers who parted from the lineages of their gurus, and still more approaches are being developed with each passing year. Some yoga styles offer greater depth than others, some involve an entire lifestyle, and others tone and sculpt your body as well as, if not better than, any other workout on the market. They all offer a way to feel better, a greater sense of well-being — whatever that means to you — and they are all valid. The bottom line is: Does the system of yoga work for you?

In writing this book I had the opportunity to interview some of the most highly regarded American yoga teachers, and while they wholeheartedly believe in the particular system they teach, the majority were quick to point out that they don't believe their style to be the *only*, or superior, approach to the practice. They have respect for all styles of yoga, and the general consensus was, as Tim Miller put it, "Do whatever it is that makes you want to do yoga." If it's Ashtanga-vinyasa yoga, the system Miller has studied for over thirty years, that's great; if not, that's fine too. Just find some way, in some form, to incorporate yoga into your life. The more people involved with yoga, on whatever level, the better. And while the yoga tradition runs the risk of becoming diluted as it expands and evolves into new systems and variations, the rewards outweigh the risks. When I asked these yoga teachers how they felt about the state of yoga in America, all but one or two of them answered with a resounding "It's great." They're pleased, even thrilled, with the fact that yoga has become so accessible, with so many styles and choices available.

In this book you will find seven core styles of yoga, plus an additional ten systems described in the "Best of the Rest" chapter. The opening of each chapter contains background information in regard to the creation, founding, and evolution of the system presented, followed by a section called "The Gist," which offers a general overview of what to expect in class if you take that style of yoga. The chapters then break down into sections, according to the main aspects and concepts of each method, to give you a clear and complete picture of that particular style of yoga. In the back of the book are resources for finding teachers and classes in the various styles.

You know yourself best. The choice of which yoga style, or styles, you want to practice is very personal and one that only you can make. Use this book as your guide. Following this introduction, on pages xiv–xv, you'll find a quick style guide for your reference. Pick a few styles that appeal to you and read through their chapters, paying attention to the subtle feelings that arise. Consider your reasons for practicing, that is, what you would like to gain from your time on the mat, and determine what type of experience resonates best with you. There's no reason to feel overwhelmed; you don't have to go out and sample every yoga class out there, nor do you have to read about every style described in this book. If something excites you, go for it and take a class. *Pick Your Yoga Practice* is meant to take you on a journey at your own pace. As your yoga practice matures, you might find yourself searching for more depth or perhaps find that your needs have shifted; when you are ready to try a new style, return to this book. Trust your gut, follow your heart, and let *Pick Your Yoga Practice* be your guide.

I wish you all the best on the journey ahead, and may our paths cross someday.

As we say in class,

Namaste.

	ACROYOGA (page 190)	ANANDA YOGA (page 170)	ANUSARA YOGA (page 184)	ASHTANGA-VINYASA YOGA (page 49)	BIKRAM YOGA (page 139)	FORREST YOGA (page 179)	INTEGRAL YOGA (page 105)	ISHTA YOGA (page 181)
Dynamic, Vigorous, and Sweaty				✳				
Heated Room					✳	✳		
Gentler Approach							✳	
Foundational for Beginners			✳					
Set Sequence of Poses				✳	✳			
Personalized Practice Provided								✳
Emphasis on Relaxation and Meditation		✳					✳	
Heavy Emphasis on Alignment			✳					
Emphasis on Strong Internal Focus		✳				✳		
Strong Ties to Traditional Indian Lineage		✳		✳			✳	
Overtly Spiritual Approach		✳	✳					
Playful Approach	✳		✳					
Emphasis on Yogic Lifestyle								
Appropriate for People with Injuries			✳			✳		✳

IYENGAR YOGA (page 65)	JIVAMUKTI YOGA (page 153)	KRIPALU YOGA (page 121)	KUNDALINI YOGA (page 81)	MOKSHA YOGA (page 187)	POWER YOGA (page 176)	SIVANANDA YOGA (page 168)	SVAROOPA YOGA (page 174)	VINIYOGA (page 172)
	❀				❀			
				❀				
						❀	❀	
❀	❀	❀						
				❀		❀		
								❀
							❀	
❀								❀
		❀	❀					
❀						❀		
	❀		❀				❀	
	❀		❀			❀		
❀								❀

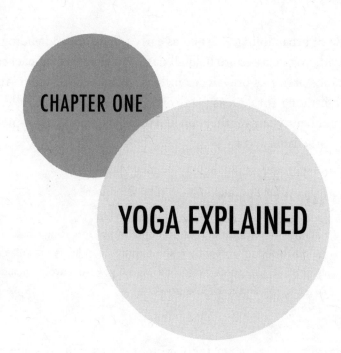

CHAPTER ONE

YOGA EXPLAINED

No longer associated with the counterculture of the 1960s, when many Americans first turned to yoga in search of a drugless high, yoga has become a nationwide cultural phenomenon and a billion-dollar industry. If you don't practice yoga, chances are you know someone who does. It seems that everyone, from athletes and celebrities to high-powered executives and politicians to stay-at-home moms and college students, is stepping onto the mat.

Modern yoga has evolved to become incredibly inclusive. Whether you're religious, spiritual, or neither, fitness-oriented or less concerned with the physical, mainstream or more eccentric, there's a yoga practice for you. Prior to the turn of the new century, yoga was never so widely available as it is today. Yoga is now offered in schools, prisons, churches, synagogues, city halls, senior centers, rehab facilities, gyms, hotels, and spas. Yoga studios have even become staples in strip malls across the country, and in large cosmopolitan cities like New York and Los Angeles, an overflow of yoga schools and centers offer sanctuary from the hustle and bustle of urban living. Starting as early as 5:30 AM and ending as late as midnight, yoga classes are held all day long, and they're packed. And while studios aren't as prevalent on the streets of small-town America, yoga is infiltrating rural areas via dedicated instructors who hold classes in small numbers wherever they can find the space. In short, people everywhere are practicing yoga.

CAN'T MAKE IT TO CLASS?

Take a class online. Yoga centers are now offering live streaming classes and classes for download to those who prefer to practice at home or on the go. With only one Google search for "online yoga," you will have a number of sites, styles, and teachers to choose from.

Americans turn to yoga for various reasons, but in some way or another they are looking to reap the practice's many benefits. They've heard yoga is good for you. They've read that yoga is great for managing stress and dealing with depression and will help them sleep better. Their doctor has told them that practicing yoga can help increase circulation, build bone mass, and lower blood pressure. They were sent by their physical therapist to cultivate postural awareness, increase range of motion, and alleviate back pain. They believed Christy Turlington when she credited yoga for her perfect bum.

Everyone, from neighbors to mothers-in-law, swears by yoga, so more and more people are taking to the mat to discover for themselves what the hype is all about. They keep coming back because the mind-body discipline works: Yoga makes you feel better. So what is it?

Yoga Explained

"What is yoga?" is a loaded question and one that could take a lifetime to answer: Ask twenty yogis, and you'll get twenty different answers. There are as many interpretations of yoga as there are Hindu gods (around 330 million). Most Americans, whether they've tried it or not, have an idea of what yoga is, even if their understanding is as rudimentary as "Yoga's that thing you do on a yoga mat when you're in yoga class that somehow involves stretching and breathing." And they are right.

Yoga is a system of exercise, but yet it's so much more. Considered a physical, mental, and spiritual discipline, yoga is an ancient belief system, a science of exploration, a process of self-discovery, a method of personal development and spiritual evolution, and an art of transformation. It is a complete approach to total well-being, and, for many, yoga is a way of life. Yoga is an all-encompassing approach to physical health, mental clarity, emotional balance, and spiritual attainment — whatever that means or looks like to you.

A PRAGMATIC SCIENCE

Originating in ancient India, yoga was developed as a pragmatic science by seers who sought answers to life's toughest questions, the type that are not easily answered: *What is the meaning of life? Who am I? Why am I here?* Through careful inquiry, experimentation, and constant observation, these seers were able to produce codified conditions that were particularly beneficial for self-realization. With a large emphasis on direct experience, such conditions became principles to help guide seekers on their individual journeys of self-discovery.

A fundamental tenet of the broader yogic tradition is that there is one universal consciousness. Call it supreme consciousness, the Divine, Brahman, God, Shiva, Buddha-nature, Allah, whatever, there is a "oneness" that encompasses everything, including you. However, we become so caught up in our individual experiences of embodied consciousness (that is, our lives) that we tend to see ourselves as separate entities operating independently from one another. Yoga, therefore, is designed to shift individual perceptions of ourselves and the world in which we live, helping us to recognize not only our inherent oneness with everyone and everything but also our union with the Divine. How that union is understood and arrived at varies from one yogic school of thought to the next (which will be explored in chapter 3), but for all intents and purposes, yoga is the method by which we realize our innate nature and highest Self inseparable from supreme consciousness and completely supported by the universe.

THE ESSENTIAL SELF

If you've read any books or articles on yoga you've probably seen the word *self* written with both a capital *S* and a lowercase *s*. In certain philosophical schools there are two selves, the lowercase self, which is associated with the material world, and the uppercase Self, your essential or transcendental Self (or spirit).

At the heart of the tradition lies the understanding that all human beings desire to belong, to be connected to something greater than themselves, to be loved. On a fundamental level all people want to be at peace and free of disease. It's safe to say that in every human heart lies an intense yearning to be happy. Yoga teaches us that these fundamental human desires are expressions of our innermost nature, that at our most basic level we are free, connected to everything and everyone, and nothing but love. We don't experience ourselves as such, because we've grown accustomed to identifying solely with our mind, which is to say our ego. Through a process of cloaking, veiling our true selves, we begin to associate with limiting self-beliefs (such as, *I'm alone, I'm not good enough, I don't deserve love*).

We practice yoga to shine the "light" on that which already resides deep in our inner consciousness, hence — en-"lighten"-ment. Practicing yoga helps clear the lenses, so to speak, taking you on an inward journey back to your deepest Self and to the realization that you have everything you need within to experience the unbounded joy and freedom that is your true nature.

YOGA IS UNION

Yoga, derived from the Sanskrit root *yuj*, meaning "to yoke" or "to bind," is most commonly interpreted to signify "union." Yoga is the process of remembering all parts of yourself, uniting your mind, heart, and spirit so that you may recognize your intrinsic wholeness and experience your own divine consciousness. Yoga is the union of self and spirit, you and God, your individual self and the quintessence of every living being and thing.

Rooted in the underlying desire for happiness, yoga is a spiritual alchemy that transforms the ordinary human conditions to generate a new state of being free from suffering. One of the great truths yoga teaches us is that joy is always available and can be experienced by simply turning within. Yoga is the practice of arriving in the present moment full of peace and grace. Every day you may feel *sukha* (fleeting pleasure) from moments of ordinary happiness arising from pleasant thoughts and experiences. The ancient yogic texts warn students against such temporary moments of joy, which are synonymous with suffering (*duhhka*) if not grounded in the larger search for the Self. Yogic wisdom tells us that you cannot experience transitory pleasures without encountering some form of suffering. Happiness that is dependent upon external conditions is never permanent, and ultimately it always causes a certain degree of pain once whatever it was that brought you joy is no longer present or new.

Beyond possessions and sensory pleasures lies a form of happiness and fulfillment independent of external circumstances. Yoga makes the bold claim that anyone can experience a profound sense of joy and ease because it is our natural way of being. Your innate Self is a joyous self. Before you began placing conditions on your happiness, before you learned to identify with whatever roles you've taken on, before the lens through which you view yourself and the world became clouded with misperception, you were inherently free, whole, divinely perfect, and happy beyond conditions. In fact, you still are at the core of your being; you merely aren't experiencing yourself as such, because you no longer identify with your true Self. In other words, if you aren't happy, something is amiss.

TODAY MORE THAN EVER

Unfortunately, people in modern society as a whole have sought happiness everywhere — relationships, material possessions, achievements, and sensory pleasures — except for deep in their heart. By taking you on an inward path, yoga becomes a transformative journey of rediscovery that makes lasting happiness possible. A great shift occurs once you understand that true joy is found within. You begin to recognize that happiness is intrinsic to the universe and that your happiness is not dependent on the impermanent conditions of the material world but originates from a deeper level of reality.

When you begin to let go of your current perceptions, realizing you are so much more than your limited experience of your body, a world full of infinite possibilities and love unfolds before you. You no longer have to look for happiness; you just *are* happy without the suffering associated with identifying with your individual ego. To have even a passing awareness of your own wholeness is to experience your innate nature, and feelings of inexplicable joy inevitably follow. Ancient seers called this happiness beyond provisional conditions *ananda*. Described as sheer, unequivocal bliss, *ananda* is not merely an emotional quality but a new state of reality that is spontaneously generated upon Self-realization. Certainly not always experienced as "joyous bliss," *ananda* can also be understood as a deeply felt sense of being okay — that no matter what happens, there's an internal knowing that everything is and always will be just fine.

The great thing about modern yoga is that you really don't need to know any of this. You don't have to desire to know your true Self or to realize your union with a higher power. You don't even have to believe in one supreme consciousness. You can simply practice yoga for the sake of practicing it, because you like it, and that is enough; the teachings of yoga say you're more than welcome to come along. But be warned, if you practice yoga long enough, small, incremental changes will begin to take place. You will most likely start living your life with more awareness, conscious of your inner motives and desires. You may begin to look at your life in different ways, and priorities may shift as a result. Your yoga will very likely seep into your relationships and how you choose to interact with the world at large.

Most important, yoga offers you insight into your own nature, giving you the tools necessary to understand yourself (and your unconscious tendencies) on a very deep level. With time and dedicated practice, yoga tends to shift what you identify with, who you experience yourself to be, and how you relate to yourself and others. Because truth be told, while yoga holds the promise of enlightenment, some of us just want to spend time on our mat, in our body, away from the stresses and challenges of everyday life. And if that helps us live our lives with a little more ease and compassion, a bit more clarity, and a lot more joy, then we are receiving the true gifts of yoga.

The Physical Practice of Yoga

In Western society, yoga has become synonymous with taking classes, doing yoga poses, and sweating; however, as we've just discussed, yoga is about so much more than developing strength and gaining flexibility. Having a healthy, strong, and toned body is the foundation for the personal growth and development yoga brings about. The physical practice of yoga postures, which is known as *hatha* yoga, is just a small window into the vast, comprehensive yoga tradition; it just happens to be the window through which most Westerners are introduced to yoga.

However, there are many branches, or practices, of yoga, including meditation, chanting, devotional prayer, and selfless service, as well as scriptural study and self-study. Taken separately or combined, they are all considered paths of spiritual development designed to elevate consciousness by helping seekers transcend conditional reality and directly experience themselves as supreme consciousness.

THE SIX MAIN BRANCHES OF YOGA

RAJA YOGA is known as the royal or king (*raja*) path of yoga as expounded in Patanjali's Yoga Sutras. Also called ashtanga yoga (the eight-limbed path), *raja* yoga is concerned with controlling the mind's activities, through concentration and meditation, for Self-realization to spontaneously occur.

BHAKTI YOGA is the path of devotion, emphasizing devotional love for and surrender to God. *Bhakti* yoga practices include daily prayer and worship, chanting the various names of God, and ornate temple rituals.

JNANA YOGA is the path of wisdom and knowledge (*jnana*), involving disciplined study of the ancient yogic scriptures and constant inquiry into the nature of self. Requiring a strong will and intellect, *jnana* yoga dissolves the veils of ignorance for the seeker to realize his or her true Self.

KARMA YOGA is the path of selfless action, the yoga of doing. Remaining completely detached from the outcome of their actions, *karma* yogis are in continuous service to the betterment of all beings with no intention of personal gain.

MANTRA YOGA is the yoga of sound. Considered sacred utterances, or sound vibrations embedded with psychospiritual energy, *mantras* are words, phrases, or simply syllables that express an attribute of divine consciousness. *Mantra* yoga involves the repetition of *mantras*.

HATHA YOGA is the yoga of force, or forceful yoga. It is the path of using the body as a vehicle for spiritual transformation.

The majority of yoga being practiced in the West is *hatha* yoga, involving *asanas* (yoga postures), *pranayama* (breathing practices), *kriyas* (internal cleansing techniques), *bandhas* (muscular locks and contractions), and *mudras* (hand gestures and seals), to greater or lesser degrees depending on the system of yoga. Often mistaken for its own style, *hatha* yoga is a general term that implies the physical practice of yoga. Ashtanga yoga, Iyengar yoga, Kripalu yoga, Jivamukti yoga, power yoga, and so forth are all practices of *hatha* yoga (though many of them also involve the other branches of yoga).

Although a physical practice, *hatha* yoga is more than a workout routine. *Hatha* yoga is a highly refined system of holistic health and well-being, addressing all layers of the self, which are not separate but interrelated, affecting one another. If the body is sick, the mind, heart, and spirit are all diminished, and vice versa; if the heart is depressed, the mind, spirit, and body are lethargic; and so forth. Considered a science with sophisticated techniques and practices, *hatha* yoga effectively balances and strengthens every system of the body — the musculoskeletal, respiratory, circulatory, digestive, nervous, and endocrine systems — allowing practitioners to release tension, increase circulation, eliminate toxins, and restore natural health and vitality.

Although the Sanskrit term *hatha* means "forceful" or "intense," when broken into its syllables, *ha* for "sun" and *tha* for "moon," it implies a joining of opposites. Masculine qualities such as strength, activeness, aggression, hardness, and heat are associated with the sun, and feminine qualities such as softness, passivity, gentleness, nurturance, and coolness are associated with the moon. The yoga of the sun and moon, *hatha* yoga, seeks to balance the opposing forces: masculine and feminine, hard and soft, right and left, inner and outer, doing and being, yin and yang. Physically *hatha* yoga requires balanced action. Through the practice we develop a balance between strength and flexibility while learning to navigate the subtle dance between effort and surrender. The neat thing is that some postures, such as forward folds, cool the body and calm the nervous system, while others, such as backbends, heat and energize the body. Then there are twists, which are referred to as "smart" poses that will either cool or heat the body, whichever is necessary to bring the body back to neutral.

The *asanas* as a whole work to restore and maintain a flexible and toned spine. For mammals, it's important to move the spine in all directions in order to keep the spinal column supple and mobile. (Ever witness a dog or cat waking up from a nap? They move, stretch, bend, and curl their spines in every direction.) The spinal column is made up of a number of vertebrae and spongy, fibrous disks that serve as spacers in between. It houses the spinal cord, which connects to the brain and, together with it, composes the central nervous system. Nerves then branch out from the spinal cord through the spaces between the vertebrae, connecting specific body parts — glands, organs, and so forth — to the brain.

THE SUBTLE BODY

Hatha yoga was also designed to address the subtle, or astral, body. According to the ancient yogic texts, seventy-two thousand energy channels, called *nadis*, exist throughout the body and correspond to the central nervous system. *Prana*, or life-force energy, runs through the *nadis*, regulating all the living functions of the body. When *pranic* energy does not flow freely through the body — which is the case when you have a rigid spine — the body, as well as the mind, can't function optimally, causing dis-ease.

Over time, with gravity, the spine begins to compress, losing space between the vertebrae and compromising the vertebral disks. The result is often an impinged nerve, cutting off the flow of energy and nerve impulses through the body, causing weakened organs and loss of muscle function, not to mention pain. Therefore, the importance of a supple yet toned spine cannot be stressed enough. The many different yoga poses flex, twist, curve, lengthen, and open the different regions of the spine, maintaining the health of the entire spinal column and strengthening the nervous system.

The Yoga of Breathing

Breath awareness is the cornerstone of any *hatha* yoga practice. Yoga is about becoming quiet, paying attention, and listening to your body. If the breath is shallow and rapid, the mind is erratic and the nervous system is destabilized, making it nearly impossible to be fully present on your mat. Take a deeper, fuller breath, and you immediately feel calmer and clearer. Conscious breathing stills the mind and draws your attention inward, allowing you to become increasingly aware of your inner experiences — the thoughts and emotions, sensations and currents of energy, tendencies and habitual patterns that arise throughout practice. You become more present, more sensitive, and more in control of your immediate experiences (responding thoughtfully rather than reacting rashly). Since the breath is the constant, serving as an anchor for your practice, anytime you catch your mind wandering off, the easiest way to become present once again is through the breath. Conscious breathing is what makes yoga a mental and spiritual discipline; without your awareness of the breath, your yoga practice is simply another form of Eastern calisthenics.

WHY THE NOSE?

The conscious yogic breathing is done in and out through the nose for multiple reasons. For starters, mouth breathing is short, rapid, and shallow, stimulating the fight-or-flight response, while nostril breathing slows the breath rate down, allowing for a fuller, deeper inhalation and a more complete exhalation. Second, both nostrils are lined with a mucous membrane that keeps the air moist, warding off infection, as well as with tiny, hair-like cilia that clean and filter the incoming air; the throat is also lined with a mucous membrane, but breathing through the mouth dries it out, reducing its protective quality. Therefore, breathing through the nose is always more optimal and actually more natural. While breathing through the nose may be difficult at first, we are designed to breathe that way, and nose breathing will become more normal with continued practice.

Aside from quieting the mind, the breath can also have powerful recuperative qualities elsewhere in the body. The full diaphragm breathing that is done in yoga (through the nose) brings more air into the lower lobes of the lungs, where the majority of the lungs' blood supply awaits the delivery of oxygen. When the breath does not reach the lower lobes, coming into contact with only the lungs' upper lobes, such as what happens with shallow mouth breathing, the heart has to pump that much harder to supply the lungs with the necessary amount of oxygen for gas exchange.

Additionally, the lungs' lower lobes contain many of the nerve receptors of the parasympathetic nervous system (the calming half of the autonomic nervous system, responsible for rest and digestive activities in the body). Deep breathing, which requires a heightened awareness, brings more oxygen into the nerve receptors located in the lower lobes of the lungs, stimulating the parasympathetic nervous system. Conversely, the nerve receptors of the sympathetic nervous system are housed in the upper lobes. Short, shallow breathing engages that part of the nervous system, triggering the fight-or-flight (stress) response; the heart beats faster, muscles tense, and blood pressure and sugar levels go up — all necessary in the face of immediate danger but very harmful if sustained. When the parasympathetic nervous system takes over, your heart rate slows, muscles release, blood pressure lowers, and so forth, inducing an overall state of relaxation and rejuvenating many of the body's systems. Therefore, your yoga practice not only helps combat mental anxiety but helps you recover and heal from the negative effects of stress as well.

On the subtle, or energetic, level, the full yogic breath brings more *prana* into the body while also regulating the life-force energy. *Prana* is the body's subtle energy. It is the animating force behind every atom, cell, organ, and system of the body, coordinating every bodily activity from the pumping of the heart to the elimination of waste. *Prana* also greatly influences the mind's state. Unstable *pranic* energy causes the mind to become agitated and the body's various systems to be irregular, producing dis-ease in the mind and body. The breath is an extension of *prana*. The deeper you breathe with conscious awareness, the more *prana* you receive. You can even direct the flow of *prana* into specific areas of the body just by sending the breath there. Furthermore, when inhalations and exhalations are equalized, *prana* becomes steadier and the mind calmer, and all the body's living systems function more optimally.

THE UNIVERSAL SOUND

Traditionally chanted at the beginning and end of class, *om* is the oldest and most widely recognized *mantra*, or sacred utterance, in the yoga tradition. The one-syllable *mantra* is pronounced in three sounds *A-U-M*, beginning in the lungs, moving through the throat, and ending in the lips, with the echo of the nasalized *m* sound hummed and then followed by a sweet, silent pause.

Symbolizing the Absolute, *om* is said to be the primordial sound of the universe — the transcendental resonance that brought everything into creation — which continues to reverberate through eternity. Scientists have now proven what the ancient seers knew: that the entire universe is pulsating in and out. Nothing exists that is not moving. Every atom is in constant pulsation, resounding a rhythmic vibration throughout the universe that is the sound of *om*.

The symbol for *om* and the sound itself represent the four basic states of consciousness: waking (*A*), dreaming (*U*), sleeping (*M*), and transcendental. The echo of the nasalized *m* sound is considered to be the fourth component of *A-U-M* and represents supreme consciousness in its unmanifested form, which is symbolized by the dot above the crescent; the three curves (and their coinciding sounds) represent manifest states of supreme consciousness.

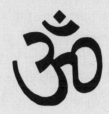

The Overall Picture

Very few students begin practicing yoga with overt spiritual ambitions. They simply want to feel and move better in their body. However, it doesn't matter whether or not your initial intentions are purely physical. What's important is that you're in your body, consciously moving and breathing, establishing a stronger mind-body connection, and cultivating a little self-awareness. Intentionally or not, you begin a process of personal growth and transformation just by practicing yoga. You might even say that yoga is for the people who are open to change, and the ones who want to stay exactly the same don't stay with yoga for very long. Your yoga practice will shift you in some way on some level, if not on all levels. In addition to helping the body gain strength and flexibility, a steady practice helps build concentration, create emotional balance, and cultivate positive qualities, such as compassion, patience, joy, and confidence.

IS YOUR YOGA WORKING?

The true measure of your yoga practice isn't whether you can do more advanced postures but rather how you treat others and yourself, the kind of person you are, and the life you lead. Progress is measured by your ability to be present to and conscious of all aspects of yourself, how well you respond rather than react impulsively, your willingness to help others, how happy you are, and more markers along those lines. You could be an amazingly adept *asana* practitioner but not a very kind person, which indicates your yoga practice isn't working for you.

During class you will experience profound moments of stillness, even if only for a few seconds at a time. The full yogic breathing helps quiet the analytical mind, which never seems to stop weighing options and considering consequences, finally allowing the intuitive mind to have a voice. The internal awareness and mental clarity cultivated in yoga help you realize certain things about yourself and your life. Over time you become skilled at recognizing that which no longer serves you — the relationships, default tendencies, reactions and other thought patterns, and roles that don't contribute to your overall happiness.

In fact, your yoga practice will typically have an interesting way of creeping into your life off the mat as you become more aware of how you feel and increasingly conscious of the choices you make. Yoga doesn't require you to change your lifestyle overnight or conform to any outside standards, but you naturally begin to gravitate toward feeling better, making better decisions and choices in your eating and lifestyle habits (and no, that doesn't mean you have to become a vegetarian to practice yoga).

You may also notice that your yoga practice is a microcosm for your life. The way you are on your mat — how you respond to challenges, handle disappointment, and relate to yourself, how present you are, how willing you are to try new things — is the way you'll be *off* your mat as well. In yoga, you get to "practice" being the way you want to be in a safe, contained environment. (After all, yoga practice is just that, practice.)

Therefore, when you are practicing, attitude is everything, as it is in life in general. To begin with, your overriding intention for practicing must be rooted in something more meaningful than external appearances or physical achievements, or your *asana* practice runs the risk of becoming just another outlet for ego gratification, and you've missed the bigger, overriding message of yoga. That means your intention for practicing doesn't necessarily have to be god-consciousness or Self-realization (although that's a good intention) but rather can and perhaps should be something personal, whether that is to feel better overall, learn more about yourself or foster self-acceptance, become a better mother or spouse, be more present or experience more joy, cultivate more peace, clarity, or ease in your life, whatever — something more meaningful than having a tight bum or being able to do the splits. Wanting to achieve an advanced posture isn't wrong; in fact, the desire can increase your dedication and drive. However, it shouldn't be your *only* reason for practicing. What if you never nail the pose? Then what? Without a higher intention, it's easy to become defeated.

Yoga is in the business of self-acceptance and exploration, which by definition can have no expectations. Sometimes you'll step onto the mat only to discover your body isn't on board to practice at the level you were hoping it was. And that's okay. In fact it's better than okay; you get to practice listening to your body and doing what's best for you in the moment. Yoga gives you permission to give yourself a break.

Of course, in a class setting it's easy to become caught up in comparing (joy's most brutal thief). As easy as it is to compare yourself to others and feel less than, it's just as easy to compare yourself and feel more than, or somehow superior, when you can "outperform" the other students in class. As you advance in your *asana* practice, it's crucial to remain humble with an open attitude and a beginner's mind. With a beginner's mind, you enter each yoga posture with the excitement and eagerness of a first-time practitioner, gently exploring new ways of aligning or moving your body in and out of the postures.

BEGINNER'S MIND

Having a beginner's mind is the Zen Buddhism concept of *shoshin*, referring to an attitude of openness, eagerness, humility, and lacking preconception, as a beginner would have, regardless of how advanced you've become in your studies. In his book *Zen Mind, Beginner's Mind*, Zen teacher Shunryu Suzuki states, "In the beginner's mind there are many possibilities, in the expert's there are few."

Conclusion

Hatha yoga has evolved over the past century to become more inclusive and continues to evolve as new scientific discoveries are made in the fields of kinesiology, psychology, neurology, and holistic health. Whichever style you practice, yoga has the ability to bring balance, physically, mentally, and emotionally, to all areas of your life. In many cases it's the only hour and a half when students don't have to think about their jobs and other worldly demands. It might be one of the few times when you don't have to consider anyone's needs but your own, so give yourself permission to remain completely present for the length of class, leave all your worries and responsibilities with your shoes at the door, and be with yourself in your body on your mat.

CHAPTER TWO

AMERICA'S YOGA HISTORY

While yoga is most commonly said to be a five-thousand-year-old tradition, its actual date of origin has been the topic of much scholarly debate. It's impossible to know exactly how old yoga is, and determining its age actually depends on what qualifies as yoga. Modern yoga, the context in which we practice yoga *asana* today, can't be more than a hundred years old; furthermore, it wasn't until the 1966 publication of B. K. S. Iyengar's book *Light on Yoga* that *hatha* yoga began to gain momentum as a movement in the West. But modern yoga is only the latest incarnation of an extremely vast tradition that has expanded and evolved through the millennia.

Ancient Indian Roots

On the basis of archaeological evidence and etymological studies, most contemporary scholars agree that yoga's roots can be traced back to the Indus Valley Civilization between 3000 and 1500 BCE on the Indian subcontinent. Throughout the region, thousands of terra-cotta seals have been unearthed depicting animals, plants, and mythological creatures, many of which are seated in postures reminiscent of traditional yoga poses. One in particular, the Pashupati Seal, portrays a horned figure surrounded by sacrificial animals sitting in a position very similar to the lotus pose. The seal is believed to be a symbol of the Hindu god Shiva. But these seals alone aren't enough to convince historians that yoga was present in the Indus Valley; the most poignant evidence of yoga's earliest existence is contained in the Vedas, the oldest scriptures on earth, produced by the Sanskrit-speaking Aryans responsible for the flourishing civilization of the time. It is in the Rig-Veda, the eldest and most important volume of the four Vedas, that yoga first materializes as a loose, unsystematic collection of beliefs and practices.

Composed of 10,600 verses and 1,028 hymns, the Rig-Veda contains a number of passages that reference protoyoga ideas and concepts, such as the belief in a singular, omnipresent being and the surrender of the ego-self, as well as practices such as concentration, austerity, accurate recitation, devotional invocation, and breath regulation. All four Vedas (*veda* meaning "wisdom") are considered revelatory texts, the hymns themselves being sacred revelations bestowed on ancient seers, known as *rishis*, during times of deep contemplation. Through the *rishis'* personal efforts and self-discipline, profound moments of insight came in the form of visions, and the illumined seers were able to "see" a true reality beyond the physical world and the confines of the conditioned mind. Referring to themselves as poets (*kavis*), the ancient seers composed thousands of hymns illustrating their sacred visions and praise for a higher power, the eternal Being (*sat*). The *rishis* then shared their revelations of a luminous reality that exceeds the limited experience of the mind with the entire Indus Valley Civilization through their poetry, the Vedas.

The ancient scriptures offer historians a window of insight into the daily and spiritual life of the highly ritualistic Indus Valley Civilization. While the ancient seers sought enlightenment, the thousands of hymns and chants contained in the Vedas basically served as instruction manuals for the various fire ceremonies and sacrifices central to the civilization's religious practices. Vedic priests, known as Brahmins, were called upon to perform public and private rituals petitioning various deities to ensure success in worldly matters such as marriage, fertility, birth, death, war, and so forth. Over time, the emphasis on ritualistic sacrifice overshadowed the higher spiritual attainments and luminous visions of the *rishis*.

FIRE RITUALS

Sacrificial fire ceremonies, known as *yajna*, were an integral part of Vedic culture. Performed by Brahmins, who chanted hymns and *mantras* to invoke a specific deity or deities, public fire rituals were held regularly for all types of occasions, calling on the favor of the various Vedic gods — one of the most important being Agni, the god of fire. Agni, who is also the acceptor of sacrifices, serves as a messenger between mortals and the other deities. Along with the recitation of *mantras* and prayers to the gods, ghee, flower garlands, and grains were also offered through Agni's fire, as Vedic priests chanted *svaha*, meaning "hail" or "oblation" as it appears in the Rig-Veda.

Toward the end of the Vedic period there was a radical shift in thought from "how" to "why" with the appearance of the Upanishads (the revelatory texts affixed to the end of the Vedas). Expounding on the essence of the Vedic scriptures, these later texts had more of a philosophical bent, in which personal inquiry and contemplation superseded the performance of rituals. The performance of Vedic rituals had required Brahmin priests, but the Upanishads marked a reorientation of power from the priests to laypeople — believing that the individual has everything he or she needs within to become Self-realized and therefore needs nothing from the world at large. Fire sacrifices and ceremonies were no longer necessary, because the Divine could be worshipped solely in the devotee's heart and mind. Seekers became renunciants who refused to play by society's norms; emphasizing complete autonomy and severe austerities, they became outcasts living in isolation. The search for the true Self became an internal spiritual journey, and meditation became the primary practice of Upanishadic sages seeking transcendental knowledge.

While the Vedas are full of esoteric passages alluding to yogic ideas, the first explicit signs of yoga's fundamental principles and practices, though embedded in profound symbolism, appear in the early Upanishads. These later scriptures fully articulate the doctrine of an ultimate reality and the transcendental Self. However, unlike the Vedic *rishis,* who shared their hymns with the ritualistic Indus Valley Civilization, the Upanishadic sages guarded the hidden knowledge of the Upanishads more closely. The word *upanishad* means "to sit down near," and a seeker had to become an initiated disciple of a Self-realized sage before receiving the profound teachings, which were passed verbally from teacher to student, establishing the oral tradition of yoga.

ORAL TRADITION

For thousands of years yoga was an oral tradition, making it nearly impossible to know its exact date of origin. Yogic teachings and practices were verbally passed from Self-realized guru to initiated disciple, beginning with the Upanishads. Students were expected to approach the teacher with the appropriate respect and humility before being invited to sit and listen; then the wisdom of the Upanishads was whispered rather than made public. Many of the sacred texts that are now available in multiple translations, including the Yoga Sutras of Patanjali, weren't written down until hundreds, and in some cases thousands, of years after they were composed.

Yoga's Epic Period

Following the writing of the Upanishads, the Indian subcontinent burgeoned with diverse threads of spiritual beliefs during a period historians have coined the Epic Age (500 BCE to 200 CE). The Upanishads mark the adoption of yogic concepts into Hinduism (Vedanta) at the same time that aspects of yoga principles and practices were implemented into the traditions of Jainism and Buddhism. Meanwhile, the sacrificial ritualism of the Orthodox priesthood was still an integral part of daily life. Ancient India was a hotbed of spirituality, and the period is responsible for India's most famous epic poems, the Ramayana and the Mahabharata, which are indeed pertinent to the study of yoga's rich history. However, the most loved and celebrated yogic text is the Bhagavad Gita, embedded in the sixth book of the Mahabharata.

The Mahabharata, composed of eighteen books (seven times the length of Homer's *Iliad* and *Odyssey* combined), is the saga of a familial feud between the Pandavas and the Kauravas over the rightful ownership of the Kuru kingdom. What ensues is an eighteen-day war between the cousin tribes, essentially understood as the struggle of good versus evil, climaxing in the Bhagavad Gita. However, as integral as the Gita is to the story told in the Mahabharata, the text is often studied as an independent work for its significant philosophical contribution to the yoga tradition.

THE GITA AND AMERICAN LITERATURE

Since the first English translation of the Bhagavad Gita, by Charles Wilkins in 1785, you can find traces of the yogic text in some of American literature's most revered works. Most notable is Ralph Waldo Emerson's poem "Brahma," which appeared in the inaugural issue of the *Atlantic Monthly* in 1857. Emerson and his Transcendentalist posse, particularly Henry David Thoreau, who declared himself a yogi to a friend in 1849, were greatly influenced by Indian thought and spiritual texts, especially the beloved Gita. After reading Wilkins's translation in 1843, Emerson wrote what became the opening lines of "Brahma," to be finished over a decade later.

Consisting of seven hundred verses, the Bhagavad Gita, whose name means "lord's song," illustrates the immortal conversation between Arjuna and his teacher, Lord Krishna, that takes place on the battlefield moments before the start of the battle. A famed archer, Arjuna is one of the five Pandava princes whose duty it is to wage war against the Kauravas and restore moral order to their kingdom. Arjuna, in a moment of hesitation while standing across from his family, teachers, and friends, proclaims that he does not wish harm to those he once loved and begins to question his duty as a soldier. Despite the moral and lawful implications of war, Lord Krishna argues that Arjuna must carry out his *dharma* (the overriding duty he has been placed on this earth to fulfill) in service of the highest good. He then imparts the lessons of the Bhagavad Gita, which include the nature and reality of humanity, the purpose of mortal life, the idea of right, or dutiful, action, and complete surrender to the lord — presenting three main approaches (or branches of yoga), *jnana* yoga, *karma* yoga, and *bhakti* yoga as a unified path to be lived daily.

Yoga's Classical Period

During the first centuries of the Common Era a variety of yoga schools existed on the Indian subcontinent; however, around 200 CE an adept yogic scholar named Patanjali systematized the fundamental elements of the yoga tradition to become its greatest authority. In 196 aphorisms, known as the Yoga Sutras (*sutra* meaning "thread"), Patanjali provided a theoretical framework for yoga theory and practice.

The 196 *sutras* of the long-renowned Yoga Sutras are organized into four chapters, or books, known as *padas*: Samadhi-Pada (the chapter on ecstasy), Sadhana-Pada (the chapter on the path of realization), Vibhuti-Pada (the chapter on powers), and Kaivalya-Pada (the chapter on liberation). Patanjali starts by simply stating, "Now begins the study of yoga," in the first *sutra*, and the second *sutra* clearly asserts the purpose of yoga according to Patanjali: *"Yoga chitta vritti nirodhah"* (Yoga is the cessation of the fluctuations of the mind). He then goes on to describe how the mind works, namely, how human beings can liberate themselves psychologically, emotionally, physically, and spiritually in this lifetime. The aim of the Yoga Sutras is *samadhi*, or spiritual equanimity. In the second chapter of his Yoga Sutras, Patanjali outlines an eightfold path called *ashtanga* (again, meaning "eight limbs"), which leads to the deeply penetrating meditative state of *samadhi*. Sometimes referred to as *raja*, or royal, yoga as well as classical yoga, Patanjali's *ashtanga* formed the foundation of the majority of yoga styles in the West.

DUELING WORLDS

According to classical yoga, which will be discussed in more depth in chapter 3, two realities are at play in the world: the relative reality of nature, which includes all aspects of manifested life, and the infinite reality of spirit, or pure consciousness. In order to realize yourself as pure consciousness, which is to say, to become enlightened, you must first become liberated from all aspects of physical nature, including your mind, body, and emotions.

Yoga's Postclassical Period

While Patanjali's classical yoga, which is based on the belief that spirit is separate from the human form, emphasized meditation and liberation from the physical dimension of life, yoga took a significant turn with the spread of *tantra* throughout India during the fourth and fifth centuries. Whereas earlier yogis paid little attention to the physical body, except to prepare it for long hours of seated meditation, now the body itself became revered as the temple of the Divine. Yogis began experimenting with and exploring the vast potential of the human body, believing the Absolute could be experienced in and through the body — thus rejecting Patanjali's dualistic worldview, which called for liberation from all aspects of a physical nature.

YOGA FOR THIS LIFETIME

Yoga's Postclassical Period was marked by the departure from Patanjali's dualistic worldview and an increase in many branches of yoga, such as *tantra, hatha,* and *kundalini* yoga. No longer seeking liberation from reality, postclassical yoga focused on the present: how to accept and live in the moment and reach your full potential in this lifetime.

Yoga's Postclassical Period, which began toward the end of the first millennium CE, was fertile ground for the emergence of *hatha* yoga.

Arising from the *tantra* movement, *hatha* yoga originally appeared around 1000 CE and is considered quite young in the larger context of the yogic tradition. In its earliest stages, *hatha* yoga was oriented toward attaining supernatural yogic abilities, known as *siddhis*, as well as achieving physical immortality. *Hatha* yogis sought to transform their body through intense and determined effort (again, *hatha* meaning "intense" or "forceful"). Like *tantra* yogis, they were interested in the interplay of opposites, believing that the cause of suffering, such as separation, delusion, and pain, was the result of polarities created in the manifest world. As discussed in chapter 1, *hatha* (*ha* meaning "sun" and *tha* meaning "moon") implies a union of opposites. Concerned with the dynamic play of energies, *hatha* yogis strove to metamorphose the physical body into the subtle body, thus attaining union with the Divine in this lifetime.

A yogi named Gorakhnath is credited with synthesizing *hatha* yoga, which also includes elements of alchemy, Buddhism, and Shaivism, around the twelfth or thirteenth century (although some scholars believe he may have lived in the eleventh century). The eldest and most important *hatha* yoga scripture is the Hatha-Yoga-Pradipika, written by the Gorakhnath disciple Swami Svatmarama sometime in the fourteenth or fifteenth century. The classic Sanskrit text includes instructions on *asana*, *pranayama*, *mudras*, *bandhas*, *chakras* (energy centers), and meditation, stating that the purpose of *hatha* yoga is to awaken *kundalini* in the subtle body and, through the advancement of *raja* yoga, reach *samadhi* (deep inner absorption).

Yoga's Inception in the West

"Sisters and brothers of America," Swami Vivekananda began his first public speech on September 11, 1893, at the Chicago World's Fair, inspiring a thunderous standing ovation from the audience of nearly seven hundred thousand attendees. Invited to join the first historical gathering of delegates representing the world's many faiths, Vivekananda brought the message of great yogic masters to the World Parliament of Religions, introducing yoga to the West for the first time. Having learned from his guru, Sri Krishna, that all faiths "are but various phases of one eternal religion," Vivekananda spoke of tolerance and the universality of consciousness on that momentous day in 1893. He presented yoga as a tool for transcending ordinary states of consciousness and arriving at the realization of our innate oneness with everything and everyone in the world. Many scholars view Vivekananda's speech as marking the end of the Postclassical Period and the beginning of modern yoga.

Before leaving India for the world's fair in Chicago, Swami Vivekananda wrote, "In America is the place, the people, the opportunity for everything new." He spent three years touring the country, giving lectures on Vedanta yogic philosophy, earning high praise from the American press, who dubbed the energetic swami the "cyclonic monk." In 1894, less than a year after arriving in the United States, he established the Vedanta Society of New York. Once back in India in 1897, the well-known swami established the Rama Krishna Order, which seeks to harmonize all the world's faiths in the serious pursuit of self-realization. Today nearly two thousand centers are affiliated with the Rama Krishna Order; those in the Western Hemisphere are known as Vedanta centers or societies, welcoming all students who wish to study Vedanta — the world's broadest religion. Swami Vivekananda not only introduced yoga to the West; he also ignited a phenomenon that ultimately opened the gates to a steady flow of Eastern thought into the West as more swamis followed in his path there.

An Ambassador of Light

Nearly thirty years later, in 1920, America's second well-known Indian swami, the beloved Paramahansa Yogananda, arrived in the United States to address the International Congress of Religious Liberals in Boston. The Indian delegate's presentation, "The Science of Religion," captivated his audience, and Yogananda quickly attracted a large following on the East Coast, where he originally founded the Self-Realization Fellowship (SRF) in 1920, "to disseminate among the nations a knowledge of definite scientific techniques for attaining direct personal experience of God." He spent the next four years lecturing on the practices and philosophy of yoga, meditation, and his scientific approach to god-realization. In 1924 Yogananda set out on a transcontinental tour, speaking to capacity crowds at some of the largest auditoriums in the States, eventually arriving in Los Angeles, where he established the international headquarters of the SRF the following year. The SRF has since expanded to nearly five hundred centers and temples around the world, dedicated to carrying on the celebrated swami's teachings and humanitarian work.

Yogananda's name signifies bliss (*ananda*) through divine union (*yoga*), and his teachings emphasize direct meditation methods for the realization of a Supreme Being and the liberation of the Self, as well as the underlying unity of all religions. He was the first Indian swami to make America his permanent home, staying from 1920 to 1952 and returning to India only once, in 1935, for a little over one year. He later wrote that in the first decade he spent in the West, tens of thousands of Americans attended his yoga classes, where he taught the more universally applicable approaches for attaining Self- or God-realization. But to his most dedicated students he introduced *kriya* yoga, which involves *pranayama* and advanced techniques of meditation that directly affect consciousness and energy. *Kriya* yoga continues to be taught through the SRF.

AUTOBIOGRAPHY OF A YOGI

Along with his founding of the Self-Realization Fellowship, one of Yogananda's greatest contributions to the study of yoga is his *Autobiography of a Yogi*. A spiritual classic, the autobiography has been translated into eighteen languages, has sold over one million copies worldwide, and was named one of the "100 Best Spiritual Books of the Century" in 1999.

The Grandfather of Modern Yoga

A five-foot-two-inch Brahmin from a small South Indian village is responsible for nearly all of the physical yoga practiced today. Born over one hundred years ago, Sri Tirumalai Krishnamacharya never left India, but without his contributions to the practice of *asana*, yoga would've never taken its current place in American pop culture. He is the grandfather of the modern yoga movement. Whatever style of yoga you practice, with the exception of Kundalini yoga and a few others, Krishnamacharya played a pivotal role in its development.

At the time of Krishnamacharya's birth in 1888, yoga had become nearly extinct while India was under British colonial rule. Practiced by only a small handful of yogis, *hatha* yoga had become taboo, and the general public was no longer interested in the tradition. However, by the turn of the next century, the Hindu revivalist movement began to breathe new life into India's rich traditions, and as a young man Krishnamacharya pursued many of the country's classic disciplines, including the study of Sanskrit, Indian medicine, and whatever yoga he could find by way of texts and the rare run-in with a practicing yogi. He went on to obtain degrees in logic, philosophy, music, and divinity but never received the deeper yogic education he longed for, and upon graduating from university he left society to seek out one of the few remaining *hatha* yoga masters, Ramamohan Brahmachari, who was living in a remote cave with his wife and three children.

For seven years Krishnamacharya lived with his master deep in the Himalayan forest, studying scriptures, learning *asana* and *pranayama*, attaining *siddhis*, and discovering the healing properties of *hatha* yoga. He is believed to have been the most developed *hatha* yoga practitioner of his time, mastering over three thousand yoga postures. At the end of his apprenticeship and at the request of his master, Krishnamacharya returned to modern society to marry, start a family, and teach *hatha* yoga to Indian householders. But first he had to capture the public's attention. In order to revitalize interest in the dying tradition, he began giving public demonstrations in the 1920s, performing elaborate *asanas* and *siddhis*, such as stopping his pulse and lifting heavy loads with his teeth. Living in grave poverty with his wife, Krishnamacharya would later describe that period of time as the most difficult in his life, but he was determined to honor his guru's request.

Krishnamacharya's fortune changed in 1931 when he was invited by the ruling family of Mysore, India, to teach yoga *asana* at their Sanskrit College. Shortly after, the maharaja (prince) offered the strict master his own yoga school in the palace's gymnastics hall. With his own yoga *shala* and finally earning a decent salary, Krishnamacharya was able to devote himself to teaching full-time and thus began one of the most fertile periods of his career. One of the greatest reformers of yoga, Krishnamacharya had a creative gift for taking obscure *asanas* and refining them, essentially adapting the *hatha* yoga tradition to meet the needs of modern society. The yoga master drew from a variety of disciplines, including Indian wrestling, gymnastics, and yoga, to develop vigorous sequences of yoga postures aimed at improving the physical endurance of his students (primarily young, athletic boys). Combining *pranayama* and *asana*, Krishnamacharya birthed the *vinyasa* style of practice that is so popular today.

ASHTANGA-VINYASA YOGA

In time, Krishnamacharya standardized his *asana* sequences into three series (primary, intermediate, and advanced), effectively developing his style of yoga known as Ashtanga-vinyasa. One of the master's most devoted students at the time was Pattabhi Jois, who preserved Krishnamacharya's work with few to no alterations. Virtually unknown to the West until the 1970s, Ashtanga-vinyasa has become one of the most popular styles of yoga under the influence of Jois, who traveled to America for the first time in 1975. On many more teaching trips abroad, throughout Europe, the Americas, and Australia, Jois spread Ashtanga yoga worldwide. By the 1980s, students from all over the globe were traveling to Mysore to study yoga under the renowned yoga teacher.

Through the 1930s and early '40s, Krishnamacharya's yoga *shala* flourished, but by 1947, the year India regained its independence from Great Britain, enrollment had dwindled to only three students. Government officials, with little interest in preserving the yoga tradition, replaced the royal family in Mysore, and without government aid Krishnamacharya's yoga school closed three years later. The great yoga master was forced into poverty once again, during which time he continued to study and evolve his teaching techniques in near isolation. His closest students believe that it was during this lonely time that the stern master's disposition began to soften as he developed more compassion for people with weaknesses and limitations.

He would eventually accept a teaching position at the Vivekananda College, in Chennai, India; however, this time students of all ages and abilities came to learn from the renowned yoga teacher — forcing Krishnamacharya once again to reform the practice of *asana*. Having to discover a new teaching approach, he began adjusting the poses according to the individual's capabilities. He offered variations, helping students refine and perfect various *asanas* as they became more adept. In his last decades, he designed appropriate approaches to *hatha* yoga for children, pregnant women, seniors, and the sick by dividing the practice into the three phases of life: youth, maturity, and old age. During the first phase the practice is focused on developing strength and flexibility, practice in the second phase concentrates on maintaining one's health while working and raising a family, and in the third phase the practice shifts from a physical focus to a spiritual union with God.

Based on the fundamental principle that yoga must be adapted according to an individual's changing needs, Krishnamacharya's second teaching method is known as *viniyoga* (a Sanskrit term implying differentiation, adaptation, and appropriate application) and continues to be taught by his son T. K. V. Desikachar. Having studied under his father for three decades, Desikachar has devoted over half of his life to teaching yoga and making the practice relevant, applicable, and useful to people of all backgrounds, ages, abilities, and mental capacities. In 1976 he founded the Krishnamacharya Yoga Mandiram (KYM), a nonprofit yoga and healing center in Chennai, and is one of today's most renowned authorities on the therapeutic applications of yoga. Viniyoga has since become a popular style in the United States, trademarked and popularized by Desikachar's student Gary Kraftsow, who is the founder, director, and leading teacher of the American Viniyoga Institute.

Krishnamacharya believed "yoga to be India's greatest gift to the world." A revolutionary reformer, he knew that yoga had to adapt (and must continue to adapt) to serve each new generation, or the tradition would be lost forever. He understood that yoga, like life, is never static and would continue to grow and evolve. And it has. Today there are dozens of styles of yoga that stem from Krishnamacharya's foundation. However, the essential teachings of the yoga tradition are timeless; Krishnamacharya merely made them accessible to millions.

The First Lady of Yoga

Although Swamis Vivekananda and Yogananda introduced yoga to the West, mainly in the form of concepts, religion, and meditation, Russian-born Indra Devi was responsible for bringing the practice of *hatha* yoga to the States. In 1947 she opened a studio in Hollywood, California, where she became known as the "First Lady of Yoga," attracting movie stars such as Marilyn Monroe and Mae West and the cosmetics magnate Elizabeth Arden. The celebrity exposure opened the door for the establishment of *hatha* yoga on the West Coast, and in the mid-1950s Walt Baptiste and his wife, Magaña, students of Yogananda, opened their yoga center in San Francisco.

Devi, a trained actor and dancer, moved to India in 1927 after escaping communist Russia three years earlier. A rising film star in the foreign land, she was fascinated with the country's rich culture and spirituality and in 1937 became the first female student of the modern yoga master Krishnamacharya in Mysore, India. Reluctant to admit a woman into his yoga school (Devi was also the first Western woman to set foot inside an *ashram*), Krishnamacharya subjected her to a stringent diet and difficult schedule. Determined, she met his every challenge, earning the harsh guru's respect as an exemplary student. After a year-long apprenticeship, he insisted Devi teach yoga and, over the course of several days, imparted lessons on *asana* instruction and sequencing, *pranayama*, and nutrition. She would later compile the teachings she received from Krishnamacharya into the first bestselling book on *hatha* yoga, *Forever Young, Forever Healthy* (1953). Three more books followed, all of which were widely popular among American housewives.

Although Devi taught a less dynamic approach to practicing *asana* and *pranayama* (her teaching style did not employ *vinyasa*), she was the first of Krishnamacharya's students to travel and teach yoga internationally. In 1939, prior to moving to California, she opened the first school of yoga in Shanghai, China, and in 1960 she became known as the "woman who brought yoga to the Kremlin" (where the practice was illegal at the time), after convincing authorities that yoga was not a religion. Fluent in five languages (Russian, French, German, English, and Spanish), Devi toured internationally throughout the second half of the twentieth century, traveling back to India many times, and yoga experienced a global diffusion.

DEVI'S STYLE OF YOGA

Known as Mataji (mother) to her followers, Devi taught a gentler style of *hatha* yoga that advised against straining. In 1966 she met Bhagawan Sri Sathya Sai Baba, believed to be an avatar, and became captivated with the guru's teachings, which included the highest ideals of peace, love, truth, right conduct, and nonviolence. Returning to India to study with Baba twenty-four times over the ensuing decade, Devi developed her own method, which she called Sai yoga.

She eventually made her way to Argentina in 1982 and, in her own words, "immediately fell in love with the country and its people." Devi moved to Buenos Aires three years later, where she quickly gained rock star–like status after a single television appearance. Capturing the hearts of Argentineans, yogis and nonyogis alike, Devi spread the teachings of love, peace, enlightenment, and the art of living a healthy, fulfilled life throughout the country. Although she continued to teach throughout the world, Buenos Aires was Devi's home for the last fifteen years of her life. She died in April 2002 at the age of 102, having continued to teach until the age of 99. Her legacy has been preserved through the Indra Devi Foundation and its six active yoga centers in Buenos Aires.

Gurus, *Ashrams*, and American Yogis

In the 1960s yoga experienced landmark growth across the United States. Maharishi Mahesh was leading the transcendental meditation movement, swamis were taking up permanent residency, and Richard Hittleman was introducing yoga to housewives in their living rooms. Knowing that most Americans wouldn't relate to the tradition's more esoteric concepts, Hittleman packaged yoga as an exercise that was good for you, and his nationally broadcast TV program, *Yoga for Health*, debuted in 1961, airing for a half-hour every morning on KTTV, in Los Angeles. He kept his presentation simple and practical, hoping students would eventually turn to meditation and yoga philosophy, and with this approach he was able reach the masses. Hittleman, who wrote a number of books on the subject, is believed to have introduced yoga to more Westerners than any other advocate of his time. By the mid-'60s, the *New York Times* estimated, from twenty thousand to one hundred thousand Americans practiced yoga. Hittleman's most popular book, *The Twenty-Eight Day Yoga Plan* (1969), went on to sell over eight million copies.

LILIAS, YOGA AND YOU

Following Hittleman's success, a housewife named Lilias Folan aired her own yoga TV program, *Lilias, Yoga and You*, on a local Cincinnati PBS station in 1972 and was carried nationally on PBS three years later, running until 1999. In her late thirties, she wore matching long-sleeved leotard and tights, either pink or red, and moved slowly through the postures, teaching viewers exactly how to do the poses and explaining the benefits of each pose.

While Hittleman was teaching yoga to middle America, Indian gurus were establishing their specific brands of yoga and spiritualism in the West. In 1959 Swami Vishnu-devananda, disciple of the famous Swami Sivananda of Rishikesh, founded the Sivananda Yoga Vedanta Centre in Montreal, Canada, birthing the first yoga vacation two years later. He was the author of the bestselling *Complete Illustrated Book of Yoga* (1960), which served as a guidebook for early adopters in the '60s, and went on to set up Sivananda yoga *ashrams* in the Bahamas, in eastern California, and near the Catskill Mountains in New York. Considered an authority on *hatha* and *raja* yoga, Swami Vishnu-devananda also established one of the first yoga teacher-training courses for Westerners. By 1970 there were Sivananda Yoga Vedanta centers in Manhattan, Chicago, Washington, DC, and Fort Lauderdale.

Arriving in the United States at the beginning of the decade, Yogi Amrit Desai was among those gurus responsible for popularizing yoga and spirituality in the 1960s and '70s. His Yoga Society of Pennsylvania, founded in 1966, grew to become one of the largest yoga centers in the country, with over twenty-five hundred students visiting weekly by the '70s. Desai and a few close students went on to open two more centers in Pennsylvania before opening the Kripalu Center for Yoga and Health, America's largest holistic health retreat center, in Massachusetts in the late '80s.

Also in 1966 Swami Satchidananda arrived in the States and founded Integral yoga, later opening his *ashram* in Yogaville, Virginia. Sponsored by artist Peter Max, who met Satchidananda in Paris, the swami arrived in New York earlier that same year, spreading the message "the truth is one, paths are many." His teachings emphasized harmony among all religions, selfless service, and the oneness of spirit. Three years after his arrival in the States, the swami opened at the original Woodstock in 1969, greeting the crowd as his "beloved brothers and sisters." Satchidananda went on to say, "America is becoming a whole. America is helping everybody in the material field, but the time has come for America to help the whole world with spirituality also."

CHANT AT WOODSTOCK

Following his opening talk, Swami Satchidananda taught the thousands of young people at Woodstock two chants: the first, *hari om hari om, hari hari om;* and the second, *rama rama rama rama rama rama rama ram.* The entire crowd then swayed, clapped, and chanted the *mantras* in unison.

The last guru to arrive in the '60s was Yogi Bhajan. A Sikh from Punjab (now Pakistan), Bhajan wore a white turban and had long graying hair (a look hippies could relate to). He taught Kundalini yoga, which was his own blend of Sikhism and *tantra*, to America's counterculture, selling yoga as a more fulfilling alternative to the psychedelic-induced altered states of consciousness they were chasing after. Bhajan quickly attracted a large following of young people and within two years opened over fifty *ashrams*, half of which were in the Southwest. He referred to his community of devoted students as family, which he called 3HO for the Healthy, Happy, Holy Organization. In 1994 he founded the International Kundalini Teachers Association, which still serves to unite Kundalini yoga teachers worldwide.

Modern Yoga's Greatest Influence

Although the aforementioned swamis and gurus led the spiritual movement of the 1960s and '70s, no one has influenced the widespread practice of *hatha* yoga more than B. K. S. Iyengar. Internationally acknowledged as one of modern yoga's greatest teachers, he is credited for his precision of alignment, postural modifications, and the use of props, which made *hatha* yoga accessible to students of all abilities despite physical limitations. Like Hittleman, Iyengar emphasized the health and therapeutic benefits of yoga, and his classes focused on *asana* and *pranayama*, leaving yoga's more esoteric practices to the swamis in their *ashrams*.

Born to a rural, impoverished family in 1918 during the influenza pandemic, Bellur Krishnamachar Sundararaja (B. K. S.) Iyengar suffered from multiple illnesses throughout his childhood, including malaria, typhoid, and tuberculosis, leaving the sickly child debilitated and unable to regularly attend school. He was introduced to yoga at the age of sixteen by his sister's husband, Sri T. Krishnamacharya (the grandfather of modern yoga), who was the head of a yoga school in Mysore and thought the practice might improve the young boy's health.

DILIGENT STUDENT

Unimpressed with B. K. S. Iyengar's stiff and weak body, Krishnamacharya didn't have much hope for him as far as the yoga *asanas* were concerned, but he still forced his sickly brother-in-law to attend classes twice a day. Iyengar practiced diligently, suffering from severe aches and pains, and in time began to notice his health was slowly but surely improving. However,

Krishnamacharya continued to pay little to no attention to Iyengar until he was forced to call upon him for a yoga demonstration when his star pupil had mysteriously disappeared just days before. Determined to change his guru's mind, Iyengar performed exceptionally well at the yoga *shala* demonstration, and a surprised Krishnamacharya began instructing Iyengar more earnestly, imposing a demanding yoga schedule and routine. Iyengar progressed rapidly and was soon assisting Krishnamacharya in more yoga demonstrations.

Although he considers Krishnamacharya his teacher, Iyengar had the opportunity to study with the yoga master for only a short period of time before he was sent to Pune, India, on a six-month teaching contract in 1936. Still not yet completely recovered from all his childhood illnesses (which took six years of dedicated yoga practice to achieve), the new yoga teacher was humiliated by his students, who quickly passed him in the performance of *asanas*. Iyengar also quickly realized that his guru had never imparted instructions, methods, or techniques for achieving the *asanas*. More determined than ever, he gained direct personal experience by devoting ten hours a day to his yoga practice, in order to fulfill his duties as a yoga teacher. Learning firsthand through a process of trial and error, Iyengar used his own body to perfect advanced poses with incredible precision, struggling and suffering great pains as he began to determine that there were incorrect ways to perform poses as well as safe, healthy ways. Over time, the master developed clear, systematic techniques for approaching the yoga poses. He also revolutionized the use of props to modify postures to meet his students' needs and in the years to come would develop therapeutic applications of the yoga poses to help heal ailments.

Iyengar's reputation as an effective yoga teacher spread throughout India, leading to a fortuitous meeting in 1952 with the violin virtuoso Yehudi Menuhin, who immediately became a student of the renowned yoga master. Influential among intellectual circles throughout the United Kingdom, as well as a global humanitarian, Menuhin arranged for Iyengar to travel abroad with him as his private yoga instructor two years later. With Menuhin, Iyengar visited Britain, France, and Switzerland, giving yoga demonstrations everywhere he went. Through the maestro, Iyengar met and taught several luminaries, among them the Queen Mother of Belgium, Queen Elisabeth, in 1958. Eighty-five at the time, Queen Elisabeth was determined to stand on her head and did so successfully under the great teacher's instruction. Through the dignitaries he was able to reach the middle class, and as word of Iyengar's magic spread throughout Europe, so did the popularity of yoga.

The 1966 publication of his international bestseller *Light on Yoga*, featuring about two hundred yoga poses and over six hundred photographs, immediately established Iyengar as the world authority on the performance of *asana*. The pivotal manual — which has been referred to as "the bible of yoga" for decades — attracted students from all over the world, who traveled to India to study with the yoga master. In 1973 Iyengar made his way to the United States for the first time at the invitation of one of his students, musician Mary Palmer. (Her daughter Mary Dunn would later be one of Iyengar yoga's most prominent teachers and the founding director of the Iyengar Yoga National Association of the United States.) Staying with Palmer in Ann Arbor, Michigan, he began lecturing and teaching large crowds at the local YMCA. Four years later the BKS Iyengar Yoga Teachers' Association was created, providing a structure for teacher certification, and over the next two decades Iyengar yoga associations began emerging all over the world, culminating in the International Iyengar Yoga Association in 2007. Iyengar himself was named by *Time* magazine as one of the "100 Most Influential People of the Century" in 2004.

Yoga Nation

By the 1970s yoga was everywhere. Ram Dass was touring college campuses with his book *Be Here Now*, instituting the spiritual quest as a lifestyle in the West. Bikram Choudhury was running his own yoga school in Beverly Hills, appearing on the *Tonight Show* in August 1974, and Pattabhi Jois arrived in the United States the following year, setting the Ashtanga yoga fire ablaze. In 1975, *Yoga Journal* published its first issue: three hundred typewritten copies printed and distributed through the Bay Area for a total of five hundred dollars. The magazine's founders, who included Judith Lasater, her husband, Ike, and Rama Jyoti Vernon (all students of B. K. S. Iyengar), set out to dispel misconceptions about yoga and further normalize it, running articles that stressed the therapeutic values of the ancient practice, such as "Yoga and the Endocrine System." They had no idea that the journal they had volunteered to publish would become the leading publication on the subject of yoga in the States.

However, despite how hard teachers such as Hittleman, Iyengar, and their successors had worked to promote yoga as a worthwhile exercise, its practice faded into the background as the 1980s' aerobics craze took over. Jane Fonda emerged as the fitness guru, and Americans wanted to sweat. By 1986 only an estimated 2 percent of the country practiced yoga, which had a reputation of being gentler and slower paced than what people were interested in at that time. Yoga would have to transform itself once again to regain the public's attention, this time reemerging as a dynamic, physically demanding workout.

Yoga's big comeback was sparked on the West Coast when Hollywood embraced the practice as a more mindful way to shed pounds and sculpt physique. By the 1990s everyone, from Sting to Sarah Jessica Parker to Kareem Abdul-Jabbar, was claiming to love yoga. By 1994 an estimated six million Americans had turned to yoga to increase flexibility, strength, and endurance, as well as to relieve tension and alleviate stress. By the time it was bought by Citicorp executive John Abbott in 1998, *Yoga Journal* had grown to sixty-six thousand in circulation. And in 2001 Christy Turlington, who had been practicing yoga for fourteen years, appeared on the cover of *Time* in a yoga pose.

POWER YOGA

Yoga really moved into the spotlight as a sweaty, full-body workout with the emergence of power yoga, a term coined by Beryl Bender Birch and Bryan Kest. The two American teachers were both practicing Pattabhi Jois's Ashtanga-vinyasa yoga and wanted get the word out that this yoga is indeed a strong, powerful workout.

The nation had become obsessed, and yoga became a billion-dollar industry. Once considered a fad, by 2005 yoga had become embedded in America's pop culture. The practice has come a long way from its hippie days in the States and has seen more than one incarnation. Today 15.8 million Americans practice yoga, and as more and more of us have stepped onto the mat, the ancient Eastern discipline of *hatha* yoga has become increasingly American. American yoga masters have emerged to found their own styles of yoga, drawing from the knowledge they gained while studying with their Indian gurus, to meet our evolving cultural needs and develop all-inclusive approaches.

TIMELINE: YOGA IN AMERICA

1893 — Swami Vivekananda addresses the World Parliament of Religions at the Chicago World's Fair.

1920 — Yogananda arrives in the United States and addresses the International Congress of Religious Liberals held in Boston on October 6. His talk, "The Science of Religion," is later expanded and published as a book.

1947 — Indra Devi opens a yoga studio in Hollywood, attracting movie stars, including Gloria Swanson, Robert Ryan, and Jennifer Jones; she becomes known as "the First Lady of Yoga."

1955 — Walt and Magaña Baptiste open their yoga center in San Francisco.

1958 — Swami Vishnu-devananda arrives in the United States.

1959 — Swami Vishnu-devananda establishes the Sivananda Yoga Vedanta Centre in Montreal, Canada, as well as the International Sivananda Yoga Vedanta Center.

1961 — Hittleman's *Yoga for Health* TV program airs on KTTV, in Los Angeles.

1966 — Yogi Amrit Desai founds the Yoga Society of Pennsylvania, later to become the Kripalu Yoga Fellowship.

1966 — Swami Satchidananda founds the Integral Yoga Institute and opens his *ashram* in Yogaville, Virginia.

1966 — The international bestseller *Light on Yoga,* by B. K. S. Iyengar, is published.

1969 — Yogi Bhajan arrives in Los Angeles and establishes the Healthy, Happy, Holy, Organization (3HO), along with his method of Kundalini yoga.

1973 — B. K. S. Iyengar arrives in the United States.

1973 — Bikram Choudhury lands in Los Angeles and founds the Bikram Yoga College of India.

1975 — Pattabhi Jois makes his first teaching debut in the United States.

1975 — *Yoga Journal* publishes its first issue.

1984 — David Life and Sharon Gannon found Jivamukti yoga.

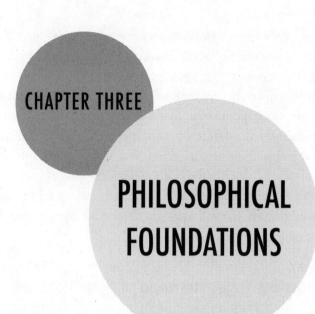

CHAPTER THREE

PHILOSOPHICAL FOUNDATIONS

Yoga is both a philosophy and the scientific application, or practices, of its philosophical vision. Through the study and application of yoga we begin to understand our experience of the universe and of ourselves, as well as our relationships to everything. How those relationships and experiences are understood varies from one school of thought to the next, according to each school's vision of how the world was created and our place in it.

YOGA IS NOT A RELIGION

Although deeply embedded in Hindu tradition, yoga is not Hinduism, nor do you have to be Hindu to practice yoga. Yoga is a methodology for personal and spiritual development, composed of different philosophical systems that prescribe a certain way of living and interacting with the world at large, with its own decree of morals, scriptures, physical postures, cleansing practices, and breathing and meditation techniques.

Today, three dominant worldviews have emerged to form the foundation of *hatha* yoga in the West: classical yoga, Advaita Vedanta, and *tantra*. Almost all modern yoga systems are rooted in one or more of these Indian schools of thought, creating context for practice and what can be very different class experiences: The worldview that a style ascribes to ultimately influences the nature of class, including the teacher's attitude, how postural instructions are delivered, and what qualities of heart and mind are emphasized. And although the presence of a spiritual philosophy isn't always overt in class, a basic understanding of the following three philosophical visions will help you determine a yoga style that supports your intention for practicing.

Classical Yoga: The Yoga of Sage Patanjali

The majority of yoga styles practiced in the West are based upon an eight-limbed yoga system, known as ashtanga yoga (*ashta* meaning "eight" and *anga* meaning "limb"), which was outlined more than two thousand years ago by the Indian sage Patanjali in his Yoga Sutras. In 196 concise aphorisms, known as *sutras*, the scholar compiled and systematized the most important principles, theories, and practices of the yoga tradition for the first time in history. By providing yoga with a codified theoretical framework, Patanjali gave the tradition its classical format; hence, the school of thought delineated in the Yoga Sutras is commonly referred to as classical yoga.

A dualistic philosophy, classical yoga draws a clear distinction between spirit (*purusha*) and nature (*prakriti*), two realms of reality that exist simultaneously but never reside together. Everything that is relative — including your body, thoughts, and emotions — belongs to the manifest, material realm of nature. Spirit, which is considered your true or highest Self, on the other hand, is infinite, absolute, and unchanging. Patanjali observed that human suffering is a result of identification with *prakriti*, an association with our body, mind, and emotions, which are not absolute. This association creates limited notions of reality and ourselves. To become liberated from this limited existence and thus free from suffering, one must transcend the material world. Since your spirit, or true Self, is absolute, forever beyond this physical realm, nature is considered an obstacle that must be overcome. You must gain complete mastery of and control over your body, thoughts, and emotions in order to isolate *purusha* from the various aspects of the physical world and for pure awareness to spontaneously emerge.

Enter ashtanga yoga. Beginning with an ethical foundation and resulting in spiritual transcendence, Patanjali's eightfold path toward enlightenment outlines specific disciplines and techniques that prepare you to realize your true Self separately from your experience of the physical world. The path is presented as an upward ladder consisting of eight successive limbs, each limb being preparation for the next, ascending from the most external physical practices (postures and controlled-breathing techniques) to the more internal practices (concentration and meditation). At each stage, from the body and breath to the senses and fluctuations of the mind, an increased level of control is attained, until the seeker has complete mastery over his thoughts and emotions. During the final stage of ashtanga yoga, the seeker is ripe for the spontaneous occurrence of isolation from *prakriti* and complete absorption into *purusha*, resulting in the ecstatic state of pure existence.

ASHTANGA YOGA

YAMA (moral discipline): Particular ethical standards, or virtues, which serve as behavioral codes for our relationships with others

NIYAMA (self-restraint): Particular observances of personal conduct dealing with physical and mental discipline, which serve as behavioral codes for our relationship with ourselves

ASANA (yoga postures): Practices to create firmness and flexibility of the body as well as to cultivate discipline and the ability to sustain focus, necessary for meditation

PRANAYAMA (breath control): Specific breathing techniques designed to calm the nervous system and quiet the mind to master *prana*, or life-force energy

Continued on the next page

PRATYAHARA (withdrawal of the senses): The practice of turning our awareness away from the outer world and external stimuli and inwardly focusing on the internal Self

DHARANA (concentration): Single-pointed focus achieved once the body has been prepared by *asana*, the mind calmed by *pranayama*, and the senses internalized

DHYANA (meditation): Unbroken concentration without an object of focus

SAMADHI (ecstasy): The ecstatic state that occurs at the peak of meditative absorption

Patanjali's yoga is often referred to as the royal path or king (*raja*) yoga, in which meditation is the central practice (Yoga Sutra 1.2: *yoga chitta vritti nirodha* [yoga is for the cessation of the mind's fluctuations]). Yoga *asana*, the third limb, is just one of the eight steps toward spiritual realization. Ultimately performed to transcend the physical experience — the body is a tool used for the realization that you are not your body at all but rather something absolute beyond relative form — *asana* was traditionally intended to prepare the body for a long period of seated meditation. (The word *asana* literally means "seat.") Once a student has advanced to the higher stages of practice, with the body now under control, performing yoga *asana* is no longer necessary. While certain systems continue to approach *asana* as a tool, emphasizing seated meditation as their main practice, most modern styles of yoga seek to integrate all limbs of ashtanga into one practice: performing *asana* with self-discipline, breath control, and unbroken concentration.

Advaita Vedanta

Considered the premiere and most influential subschools of the Vedanta Indian school of thought, Advaita Vedanta was first introduced to the West through the teachings of Swami Vivekananda, who spoke at the world's fair in 1893. Today there are numerous Advaita Vedanta societies and *ashrams* across the United States, which typically incorporate some form of *asana* into their spiritual practices, as well as a handful of popular *hatha* yoga styles founded on the Vedanta school of Indian philosophy.

VEDANTA SCHOOLS OF THOUGHT

Vedanta means "the end of the Vedas" and refers to multiple schools of thought that base their understanding of reality on the Upanishads, the last of the Vedic texts.

While classical yoga acknowledges the existence of two separate realities, Advaita (nondual) Vedanta is a monist philosophy alleging there is only one true reality, Brahman, which is absolute, omnipresent, transcendent, and eternal. Everything that is impermanent, including all perceivable differences (duality), is false. The world and all its multiplicity is considered an illusion — a flaw in perception — rooted in ignorance. There is only the One. And the One, Brahman, is your true being.

Imagine walking down a dark road when suddenly a snake appears a few feet in front of you. Deathly afraid of snakes, you freeze and cannot take one step farther. Then suddenly the clouds part, and the moon illuminates the path ahead, shedding light on the snake, which isn't a snake at all but a rope. The snake and rope analogy is often used in Advaita Vedanta to help explain the relationship between Brahman and the manifest world: Just as you conflated the snake with the rope, the universe is a conflation with Brahman, and just as the moon shed light on the snake to spontaneously reveal a rope, true knowledge sheds light on ignorance to spontaneously reveal the oneness of reality.

A central assumption of Advaita Vedanta is that we are born into bondage (the cycle of rebirths) because of this erroneous perception of the world and ourselves. We suffer because we are ignorant of our true nature and the oneness of reality. To attain liberation (*moksha*) and escape the cycle of rebirths, we must correct our perception and realize our true nature as Brahman. This implies the same belief that classical yoga advocates: Your body, thoughts, and emotions are not you at all; the real you, your transcendental Self, is something entirely different, and emotional pain is the result of identification with your manifest nature. However, Advaita Vedanta imparts that, rather than requiring a step-by-step process toward Self-realization, *moksha* requires only that you open up to the true knowledge of oneness and recognize all experiences of duality as a psychological illusion.

Jnana yoga, the yoga of knowledge or wisdom, is the main path of Advaita Vedanta. Though other yogas (*bhakti*, *raja*, *karma*, and *hatha* yoga) serve a purpose for Advaitins seeking to discover their true nature, only *jnana*, true knowledge, can lead one directly to *moksha*. Through deep inquiry and personal contemplation of the Upanishads, pure knowledge of Brahman is said to spontaneously arise.

NOT THIS, NOT THAT

The most common Advaita Vedanta practice is known as *neti neti* (literally, "not this, not this"). Either chanted or repeated in meditation, *neti neti* is a technique used to negate everything that is not Brahman.

Tantra

Following the establishment of classical yoga and Advaita Vedanta, Indian philosophical thought radically shifted, simultaneously acknowledging the existence of both realities (relative and absolute) and recognizing the supreme oneness of the universe, neither negating nor affirming the two previous schools of thought. (The word *tantra* means "weave" or "loom.") The *tantra* school of thought wove the two preceding philosophies together and then expanded them.

From a *tantric* nondual perspective there is no separation between spirit (*purusha*) and matter (*prakriti*) — everything in the universe is perceived as supreme consciousness, and yet everything, including all perceived differences, is real. *Tantra* does not deny the existence of duality, instead explaining the physical world as diverse manifestations or expressions of the Divine. Therefore there is nothing to transcend, no obstacles to overcome; every particle of the universe, every aspect of existence from the mundane to the sublime — including anything that may be perceived as negative — is pure consciousness.

THE FLIP OF A COIN

As with two sides of the same coin, there is no separation between supreme consciousness and the world of duality. On one side of the coin you have the many as one, and, on the reverse side, the one expressing itself as the many.

For Tantrikas (practitioners of *tantra*), physical existence is not a problem but instead a gift, rebirth no longer a punishment but an opportunity to experience life again, with all its bodily experiences. Because there is nothing that is not consciousness, everything and every experience is an opportunity to experience your intrinsic nature. Your physical body does not limit you. Instead it's in your body that you are able to experience the ecstatic dance of the sublime. So *tantra* has a slightly different spin on the practice of *asana*. Instead of being performed as a means to an end — a rung on the ladder to transcendence — as it is in classical yoga, *asana* practice becomes a celebration of your innate freedom in this physical form here and now.

While most people associate the practice of yoga postures with Patanjali's classical yoga (*asana* being the third limb of ashtanga yoga), *hatha* yoga didn't actually materialize until the *tantra* movement came together; therefore, some would argue that all styles of modern yoga are based in *tantra*, though their philosophies are ascribed to classical yoga.

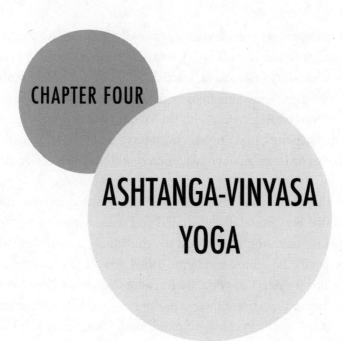

CHAPTER FOUR

ASHTANGA-VINYASA YOGA

If we practice the science of yoga, which is useful to the entire human community and which yields happiness both here and hereafter — if we practice it without fail, we will then attain physical, mental, and spiritual happiness, and our minds will flood towards the Self.

— **SRI K. PATTABHI JOIS**, founder of Ashtanga-vinyasa yoga

Introduction: Steeped in Ancient Tradition

Ashtanga-vinyasa yoga is a dynamic, physically demanding practice that synchronizes the breath with every movement to produce internal heat as students move through a set series of postures. The method is a process of purification, heating the body and eliminating toxins and impurities through sweat. Over time, the result is a healthy, toned, and flexible body — the foundation for cleansing the sense organs and controlling the mind in order for Self-realization to occur.

The classical system of yoga is accredited to Sri K. Pattabhi Jois (known to his students as Guruji), who emphasized that the "Ashtanga yoga method is Patanjali Yoga," which is to say that the popular style of yoga *is* the eight-limbed path of internal purification depicted in Patanjali's Yoga Sutras. Beginning with the *yamas* (moral code) and *niyamas* (personal discipline), practitioners must progress through all eight stages of practice in order to achieve *yoga*, union with the universal Self. However, to be able to practice the first and second limbs, the *yamas* and *niyamas*, the body must first be strong and healthy, free of disease or obstacles that may destabilize the mind and sense organs. Jois, therefore, began by first teaching his students the third limb, *asana*. With *asana* he taught a specific breathing technique called *ujjayi* breath, one of the key elements of this system of yoga. By learning to regulate their breath, students can begin to stabilize their sense organs and still their mind. With strength, steadiness, and clarity of mind, students are then able and ready to contemplate and develop the *yamas* and *niyamas* as they move into the deeper stages of yoga.

YAMAS AND NIYAMAS

In Sanskrit the word *yama* means "restraint," and *niyama* means "observances." Together they constitute the dos and don'ts involved in leading a spiritual life.

The Five *Yamas*

ahimsa (restraint from doing harm)
satya (truthfulness)
asteya (restraint from stealing)
brahmacharya (avoidance of sexual exploitation)
aparigraha (nonpossessiveness or greedlessness)

The Five *Niyamas*

shaucha (purity)
santosha (contentment)
tapas (spiritual austerities)
swadhyaya (self- and scriptural study)
ishwarapranidhana (surrender to or devotion to God)

The first four limbs of Patanjali's Ashtanga yoga, *yama, niyama, asana,* and *pranayama,* are considered external cleansing practices, and the remaining four, *pratyahara* (sense control), *dharana* (concentration), *dhyana* (meditation), and *samadhi* (contemplation), are internal spiritual disciplines. For Ashtangis (Ashtanga yoga practitioners) the purpose of yoga is to control the mind: "*citta vritti nirodhah,*" as Patanjali states in his second *sutra.* Only when the mind is quiet and focused in a single direction can the true nature of your existence, the universal Self, be revealed. Through dedicated practice and the correct application of the Ashtanga-vinyasa yoga method as presented by Sri K. Pattabhi Jois, one undergoes a process of external and internal purification that removes unnecessary stimuli and clears the mind, eventually leading to the full realization of all eight limbs of Patanjali's yoga.

THE SIX POISONS SURROUNDING THE SPIRITUAL HEART

According to Yoga Shastra (the "definitive yoga teachings"), the Divine dwells in the heart but is concealed by six poisons: *kama* (desire), *krodha* (anger), *moha* (delusion), *lobha* (greed), *matsarya* (envy), and *mada* (sloth). Jois taught that when the internal purification process is complete, which requires a dedicated and disciplined yoga practice sustained over a significant period of time, bringing the mind and sense organs under control, the six poisons burn away one by one, revealing the inner Self.

While Ashtanga yoga's philosophical foundation is rooted in the Yoga Sutras, the practical application of the method was derived from another ancient text, called the Yoga Korunta. Attributed to the sage Vamana Rishi, this source describes a precise system of *hatha* yoga, including *asana, bandhas* (body locks), *drishtis* (gazes), and most notably *vinyasa. Vinyasa,* meaning "breathing-movement system," is the linking of movement and breath (one breath for every movement) that originated with this style of yoga. With the growing popularity of Ashtanga-vinyasa yoga in the West beginning in the 1980s, teachers who started out in the traditional system have since developed their own expressions of the practice using the principle of *vinyasa*, including power yoga, Prana Flow yoga, vinyasa flow yoga, Baptiste Flow, and many others. The neat part about so many styles using the same *vinyasa* format is that once you've learned the concept you will feel comfortable in many yoga classes around the world, regardless of their title. However, there are six set series of poses taken directly from the Yoga Korunta, which is believed to have depicted groups of *asanas* (*korunta* meaning "group"), that are unique to the Ashtanga-vinyasa yoga method.

Although it's nearly impossible to prove that the Yoga Korunta ever existed, the Ashtanga yoga tradition claims that every aspect of the *vinyasa asana* method has continued to be practiced in the same manner for thousands of years. Orally transmitted, the text was imparted to Sri T. Krishnamacharya during his studies with his guru, Ramamohan Brahmachari, in the early 1900s. Having learned it by heart, Krishnamacharya then passed the system down to his oldest and dearest student, Sri K. Pattabhi Jois, who spent over twenty-five years under the guidance of the master, beginning in 1927. In time, from 1958 to 1960, Jois wrote a complete guide to the Ashtanga-vinyasa yoga method in his book *Yoga Mala*, first published in 1962, over a decade before his first visit to America, in 1975 (although the English translation of the *Yoga Mala* wasn't published until 1999). Never straying from what he had learned from his teacher, Jois taught Ashtanga yoga around the world for more than fifty years. His book, testimony that the tradition has remained unchanged over the decades, continues to serve as a reference for Ashtanga students and teachers worldwide.

Parampara, knowledge that is transmitted from guru to disciple, is an essential component of the Ashtanga yoga method. According to the tradition, only instructions that come from within *parampara* are true, effective, and complete. The style stresses over and over again the importance of practicing under the guidance of a traditionally trained teacher authorized by the Sri K. Pattabhi Jois Ashtanga Yoga Institute (KPJAYI). Students travel from all over the world to study Ashtanga-vinyasa yoga from its source at the KPJAYI in Mysore, India, where they are expected to stay for a minimum of one month. Experienced and dedicated students who continue to study at KPJAYI and demonstrate a high level of proficiency and appreciation for the traditional form of Ashtanga yoga as taught by Sri K. Pattabhi Jois may receive authorization from the institute to teach the method, ensuring *parampara* and, in that way, preserving the lineage. For Ashtanga yoga students, there is something truly magical about being part of an ancient system and tradition that has been handed down through generations of yogis.

KPJAYI-APPROVED TEACHERS

The KPJAYI does not approve of teacher training under any other name. Teachers who are authorized or certified by the institute are required to teach the method as it continues to be taught by Pattabhi Jois's grandson, R. Sharath Jois, at KPJAYI. In North America there are fewer than 150 authorized Ashtanga yoga teachers and only 19 certified. For an official list of authorized teachers worldwide, visit kpjayi.org.

The Gist: It's All about the Breath

Ashtanga yoga is very straightforward. Students practice a prescribed sequence of *asanas* in the same format in every class. Beginning with Sun Salutations and ending with Padmasana (Lotus Pose) followed by rest, there are six different series of postures in Ashtanga yoga. Within any given series, each posture is preparation for the next, cultivating the strength, flexibility, and balance for the student to move on, and the series themselves become progressively more advanced. Once a student demonstrates full understanding of one series' fundamentals and has practically mastered the sequence of poses, which can take years of dedicated practice, he or she may proceed to the next series.

The first, or primary, series in Ashtanga yoga is called Yoga Chikitsa, meaning "yoga therapy." Designed to purify and heal the body, the primary series builds strength, stamina, and flexibility while realigning the spine and detoxifying the body. The series of about seventy-five *asanas*, including standing poses, seated poses, inversions, and backbends, generally takes an hour and a half to two hours to complete and forms the foundation of all the subsequent series. Students are also introduced to the five main aspects of Ashtanga yoga in the style's first series: *ujjayi* breath, *vinyasa*, *drishti* (gaze), *bandhas*, and linking of the *asanas*. Also through the primary series, students begin to develop a consistent daily practice.

THE PRACTICE OF REFINEMENT

Working within a strict series of *asanas* can be a process that is equally frustrating and transformative. While doing the same series of poses again and again (and again and again) may be boring, within repetition lies an opportunity to deepen your yoga practice. Instead of moving on to the next series once those plateaus of boredom are reached, Ashtanga yogis seek more depth, the subtler aspects of practice beyond the external, continually refining their practice and in that way reaping its wide range of benefits. In theory, one series is enough for a lifetime of practice.

Once the primary series is strong, students can begin practicing the second, or intermediate, series (usually with the permission of their teacher). Called Nadi Shodana, meaning "nerve cleansing," the intermediate series opens and cleanses the thousands of energy channels, or *nadis*, purifying and strengthening the nervous system. Both the first and second series begin and end in the same format, starting with the six fundamental standing positions (and their variations) directly following Sun Salutations A and B and concluding with the finishing postures; however, the first series contains a number of forward folds, and the second series emphasizes backbends. For that reason, the intermediate series is an ideal complement to the primary series, and teachers will often introduce at least the first few poses of the second series after about a year of practice. By then a student has learned at least the entire first series and should be able to breathe steadily throughout it.

Traditionally taught one-on-one, guru to disciple, in increments over time, Ashtanga yoga places a lot of emphasis on learning, practicing, and advancing at one's personal pace. On the first day of class, beginning students are introduced to the concept of *vinyasa* through Sun Salutation A, followed by Padmasana (Lotus Pose), deep breathing, and a few minutes of rest. On the second day Sun Salutation B is taught after A, and the class concludes in the same manner as on the previous day (Lotus Pose, deep breathing, and rest). Once a student has learned how to properly breathe and has moved through both Sun Salutations A and B, *asanas* are consecutively introduced; once one pose has been mastered, the next is offered, until the entire series has been learned.

THIRD, FOURTH, FIFTH, AND SIXTH SERIES

The remaining four Ashtanga yoga series were originally only two comprehensive series, but Pattabhi Jois subdivided the advanced series into four series (A, B, C, and D) in order to make them more accessible to more students (although still appropriate for only very advanced practitioners). The four advanced series are known as Sthira Bhaga, which means "sublime serenity" (the reward for years of dedicated practice), and are where longtime Ashtangis integrate the strength and grace of practice, mastering difficult arm balances, hip openers, and backbends.

While the traditional method is still taught at the Sri K. Pattabhi Jois Ashtanga Yoga Institute, two main methods of teaching have emerged in the West: the self-led method, known as the "Mysore style" of practice, and the traditional counting method. In their unique approach to Ashtanga yoga, Mysore classes give students the opportunity to practice at their own pace and level of ability under the guidance of an experienced teacher. In one Mysore class, there may be fifteen students working on fifteen different postures or sections of the series, such that you may just be starting your standing poses while the person next to you is already lying down to rest. More experienced students will be able to complete an entire series of *asanas* in a single two-hour class, whereas less experienced students may need extra help from the teacher in learning the correct order of poses. The beautiful thing about Mysore-style classes is the individual attention students receive. A mature and compassionate teacher will be able to offer modifications, even show a student where he or she can leave parts of the series out, as well as how to apply the method to meet the student's personal needs.

The majority of studios also offer group-guided Ashtanga yoga classes, during which the *vinyasas* are counted aloud and the teacher leads the class in the order of poses. Rather than placing prime importance on the correct bodily alignment of each posture, Ashtanga-vinyasa yoga is a breath-centric practice. Allowed to be a little sloppy at first (within reason), new students are encouraged to focus on their breath, allowing the rest to come in time. Most Ashtanga teachers possess a come-do-what-you-can attitude, wanting new students to get used to being in their body, moving through space, and consciously breathing before honing their postural alignment, which is introduced only as practice deepens. Ultimately, "form follows function," meaning that the form of the pose will depend on the body's limitations, such as range of motion and strength. The theory is that as the body gains strength and flexibility, the alignment of the posture will become more achievable and props will be needed less often, though a skilled teacher will be able to work with a wide range of abilities and physiques, including students considered to be handicapped.

ASHTANGA YOGA *SHALA*

Traditionally called a yoga *shala* (Sanskrit for "house"), an Ashtanga yoga studio typically offers Mysore as well as group-guided classes daily, with the exception of moon days. Twice a month the *shala* is closed in observation of the full and the new moon, which are yoga holidays in the Ashtanga tradition. The phases of the moon have different energetic effects on the body: full moons are emotional and ungrounding, and new moons are dense and sluggish. By observing moon days, Ashtanga yogis honor and attune to the rhythms of nature.

Traditionally, every Ashtanga yoga practice begins and ends with an opening and closing chant. Chanted one time, in Sanskrit, the opening *mantra* pays homage to the lineage of teachers that came before, and the closing *mantra* is an offering of the effort and fruits of practice for the benefit of all beings, bringing practice to a peaceful end.

ASHTANGA YOGA OPENING AND CLOSING CHANTS

Opening Chant

om
vande gurunam charanaravinde
sandarshita svatma sukava bodhe
nih sreyase jangalikayamane
samsara halahala mohashantyai
abahu purushakaram
shankhacakrsi dharinam
sahasra sirasam svetam
pranamami patanjalim
om

om
I bow to the lotus feet of the Supreme Guru,
which awaken insight into the happiness of pure Being,
which are the refuge, the jungle physician,
which eliminate the delusion caused by the poisonous herb of Samsara
     (conditioned existence).
I prostrate before the sage Patanjali,
who has thousands of radiant, white heads (as the divine serpent, Ananta)
and who has, as far as his arms, assumed the form of a man
holding a conch shell (divine sound), a wheel (discus of light or infinite time)
     and a sword (discrimination).
om

Closing Chant

om
svasthi praja bhyaha pari pala yantam
nya yena margena mahim mahishaha
go brahmanebhyaha shubamastu nityam

Continued on the next page

lokah samastah sukhino bhavantu
om shanti shanti shantihi

om
May the rulers of the earth keep to the path of virtue
for protecting the welfare of all generations.
May the religious, and all peoples, be forever blessed.
May all beings everywhere be happy and free.
Om peace, peace, perfect peace.

Vinyasa and the Victorious Breath

Vinyasa forms the foundation of Ashtanga yoga practice. Each movement is accompanied by one breath, an inhalation or an exhalation, to create one system of breathing and moving, or one *vinyasa*. The result is a graceful flowing sequence of movements done to the rhythm of your breath. The breath and the movement are married in such a way that they enhance each other, with inhalations supporting movements that expand or lift the body or both, and exhalations supporting movements that contract or lower the body or both. For example, raising your arms up overhead on an inhalation expands the breath further; exhaling as you bend forward allows the body to fold, or contract, deeper.

Fundamental to the concept of *vinyasa* is the *ujjayi* breath, which is common to most styles of yoga. Involving long, even breaths taken in and out of the nose, the technique creates an ocean sound by subtly contracting the muscles around the glottis (the vocal folds and the space between those folds and the upper part of the larynx) as air is pulled through the back of the throat. Known as the "victorious breath," the technique regulates and expands the breath, increasing the volume of oxygen received and the amount of *prana* (life-force energy) absorbed into the body. The rhythm, sound, and texture of the *ujjayi* breath continuously draw the mind in on itself, establishing the meditative aspect of Ashtanga-vinyasa yoga practice.

To create the ocean sound of the *ujjayi* breath, start by inhaling and exhaling through the mouth, producing an *aaaahhhh* sound on your inhalation and a *hhhhaaaa* on your exhalation. After a few rounds, try generating the same sounds with your mouth closed. It's very common for beginning students to essentially sniff the air in and out of the nose in an attempt to make the ocean-like *ujjayi* sound; however, the sound originates from the back of the throat, not in the nose. (It may be helpful to lightly place a finger or two at the base of the throat and concentrate on drawing the breath in from here, as if you're pulling a rope.) The next step is to balance the length, sound, and quality of your inhalations and exhalations. Most likely, your exhalations will be longer and stronger, so you may want to focus on expanding your inhalations to match your exhalations. As you continue with your daily Ashtanga practice, you will gradually increase the intensity and length of your breaths to match some of the longer movements and transitions between poses.

UJJAYI BREATHING

Physiologically, the *ujjayi* breath is a valuable technique for cleansing the lungs. For starters, inhaling through the nose humidifies and removes dust particles from the air you're breathing in. Second, the murmuring sound of the *ujjayi* breath subtly vibrates the bronchi, activating the ciliated epithelium, which also helps remove dust particles from the lungs. Lastly, the extended exhalation greatly reduces the amount of residual air left in the lungs. Therefore, the *ujjayi* breathing technique is particularly beneficial for those suffering from asthma or chronic obstructive lung conditions.

Every Ashtanga yoga practice starts with the *vinyasa* sequence Surya Namaskar, or Sun Salutation, A. The sequence begins and ends with practitioners in Samastitihi, standing upright, centered and steady at the front of the mat, and comprises nine *vinyasas*. Each movement is counted in Sanskrit, as follows: *ekam* (one), *dve* (two), *trini* (three), *catvari* (four), *pancha* (five), *sat* (six), *sapta* (seven), *astau* (eight), and *nava* (nine). Repeated five times, the nine *vinyasas* are performed as a continuous flow without stopping or taking extra breaths in any one position, with the exception of Downward-Facing Dog (Adho Mukha Svanasana), the sixth *vinyasa*, which is held for the count of five full rounds of breath. The first

Sun Salutation flows directly into the second, Surya Namaskar B, consisting of seventeen movements, counted in Sanskrit and repeated five times. Together, the rhythmic *ujjayi* breath and repetitive movements of the Sun Salutations are very centering and generate a calm, steady state of well-being.

SALUTE TO THE SUN

Traditionally performed in the morning to greet the rising sun, Surya Namaskar is a yogic ritual worshipping the sun (*surya*) as the giver of light and life. *Namaskar* is derived from the Sanskrit root *namas*, meaning "to bow." There are many variations of Sun Salutations, and almost all systems of yoga will incorporate them into their teachings.

The last exhalation of Surya Namaskar B flows directly into the first inhalation of the predetermined sequence of postures. Every pose has its own sequence of *vinyasas*, beginning and ending with Samastitihi. Ashtanga yoga practice is often described as a garland, or *mala* in Sanskrit, the poses strung like beads upon the thread of *vinyasas* woven together by the breath. Often misunderstood, the *vinyasas* are not in-between poses; rather, the *asanas* themselves are brief pauses between *vinyasas*, creating a nearly continuous flowing sequence of movement through the entire practice.

The *vinyasas* create and maintain the necessary heat to perform the *asanas*. In the Yoga Korunta, Vamana Rishi taught, "Do not do yoga without *vinyasa*" (*vina vinyasa yogena asanadih na karayet*). The purpose of the ancient technique is to purify the body. Synchronizing the *ujjayi* breath with the fluid movements of Ashtanga yoga warms, or, as Pattabhi Jois always said, "boils," the blood — thinning and therefore cleaning it, as thick blood is known to be dirty with impurities. Thin blood circulates more freely throughout the body as you flow through the dynamic poses, easing joint pain (often a result of poor circulation) and removing toxins from the fatty layers, muscle tissue, internal organs, and glands, which are then carried out of the body by the sweat produced by the dynamic practice. The result is a healthy, strong, light, and energized body.

If you aren't sweating, you aren't applying the *vinyasa* technique correctly. You want to sweat. Sweating is the body's natural way of getting rid of impure substances. The more you sweat, the more toxins you eliminate. That being said, if you force the internal cleansing process you may become sick. The systematic method of Ashtanga yoga, with its progressive series of *asanas*, promotes a gradual purification process as students progress more deeply into their yoga practice. Once the body is purified, it's possible to cleanse the nervous system, followed by the sense organs, after which controlling the mind is easily accomplished.

Bandhas: Containers of Energy

An important component of the breathing-movement system is the application of *bandhas*, meaning "locks" or "seals," in Ashtanga yoga. While the expansive, powerful *ujjayi* breath, enhanced by the movements of *vinyasa*, brings more *prana* into the body, the *bandhas* harness and direct the life-force energy received. The Ashtanga-vinyasa yoga method uses three main *bandhas*: *mula bandha* (root lock), *uddiyana bandha* (abdominal lock), and *jalandhara bandha* (throat lock). Together the three locks also work to "unlock" even more *pranic* energy found in the various energy centers of the body, directing *prana* into the seventy-two thousand *nadis* (energy channels) of the subtle body.

Mula bandha, applied through the genital region of the body, is responsible for internally sealing *prana* in the body, drawing energy into the Muladhara (or root) *chakra* located at the base of the spine. Applied through the abdominal region, *uddiyana* (meaning "upward flying") *bandha* then pulls the energy up through the *nadis*. Both *bandhas* are an integral part of the *ujjayi* breathing technique. (Jois taught, "Without *bandhas*, breathing will not be correct and the *asana* will give no benefit.") Linked to the exhalation, *mula bandha* draws energy downward, connecting you with the element earth, which is necessary for a firm foundation; *uddiyana bandha* is linked to the inhalation, connecting you with the element air, allowing you to become lighter. When balanced, energy flows freely between the two opposing forces, helping to build a strong internal fire and giving strength, lightness, and health to the body.

Anatomically the *bandhas*, combined with the breath, help create alignment in the body by creating length in the spine and stability in the torso. *Mula bandha* is achieved by lightly drawing the pelvic floor in and up. In the beginning, it's easiest to explore the physical action of *mula bandha* on the end of an inhalation, contracting the muscles through the genital region, including the anal sphincter and the perineum, as you empty out the breath. This general action, strong and muscular at first, will become subtler with practice and increased awareness. *Uddiyana bandha* is applied by gently drawing the low belly inward, lightly activating the transverse abdominal muscles (therefore protecting the low back). Place a hand at two fingers' width below the navel at the end of an exhalation; then as you begin your next inhalation, pull the area in and up. Although both *bandhas* are to be engaged continuously throughout practice in Ashtanga yoga, this may be difficult at first. Start by exploring their actions in Downward-Facing Dog during the first Sun Salutations. Over time, you will begin to remind yourself to apply the *bandhas* more frequently until they are engaged throughout the entire practice.

DANCE OF OPPOSITES

Ashtanga yoga symbolizes the temporary cosmic dance of opposing forces as described in the *tantra* — the dance between light and dark, sun and moon, male and female, positive and negative, ascending energy (*prana*) and descending energy (*apana*), *mula bandha* and *uddiyana bandha*. Ashtanga yoga seeks to balance the opposing forces, expanding and moving upward on every inhalation and condensing and rooting downward on every exhalation, to create internal harmony.

The third lock in Ashtanga yoga is *jalandhara bandha*, which is achieved by slightly lowering the chin and often occurs naturally in various *asanas* according to the pose's *drishti* (point of gaze), or head position. *Jalandhara bandha*, or throat lock, creates a seal preventing *pranic* energy from escaping out the top of the body and is primarily used during *pranayama* (breath control) practices. However, the student is advised to practice *pranayama* with *jalandhara bandha* only under the guidance of an experienced teacher.

Tristhana: The Lotus Blossom of Ashtanga Yoga

A natural fluidity and gracefulness to the practice arises once a state of *tristhana* is achieved — the key to developing the spiritual dimensions of Ashtanga-vinyasa yoga. *Tristhana* is the union of three places of attention: synchronicity of breath and movement (*vinyasa*), tension (*bandha*), and gaze (*drishti*). Through repetition, *tristhana* is attained, and the energy carries the body with great ease through the *vinyasas* and poses, shifting the focus from the external physical practice to the internal spiritual journey.

Always performed together, *vinyasa*, *bandhas*, and *drishti* cover three levels of purification: the body, the nervous system, and the mind. *Vinyasa*, as discussed in the previous section, effectively cleanses the body; the *asanas* and the application of *bandhas* develop strength, flexibility, and balance in the body through the predetermined sequences. The long, even inhalations (*rechaka*) and exhalations (*puraka*) of the powerful *ujjayi* breath stoke the internal fire, burning away impurities and strengthening the nervous system. Meanwhile, *drishti* stabilizes and purifies the sense organs and functions of the mind.

INTERNAL FIRE

The place of fire in the body is located two fingers' width below the navel in the nerve plexus. Known as the *kanda*, it is the point where all the energy channels meet. Energy is continuously pulsating from this central point, drawing together on the exhalation and radiating on the inhalation. Long, even breaths stoke the internal fire, cleansing and strengthening the thousands of *nadis*, or nerve pathways.

Drishti is the point of focus or looking place while you are in a pose. There are nine *drishtis* in the Ashtanga yoga method: the tip of the nose, between the eyebrows, the navel, the hand, the thumbs, the toes, the sky, the far right, and the far left. Having little to do with what you are actually looking at, *drishti* is used to focus the mind and withdraw the senses, turning the gaze inward. *Drishti*, therefore, is the gateway into the internal cleansing practices of Patanjali's ashtanga yoga. By focusing the mind on a single point, students begin to develop an internal awareness, leading to the development of the sixth and seventh limbs — concentration (*dharana*) and meditation (*dhyana*) — in preparation for the attainment of *samadhi*, the final step of Patanjali's yoga.

Conclusion

Ashtanga yoga is a daily practice that requires discipline, motivation, and stamina, inspiring devoted loyalty in its students. It takes years of dedicated practice to understand the system's true essence, and longtime Ashtanga yoga teachers emphasize that the practice is a journey meant to support you for a lifetime. While the dynamic style promotes physical strength and athletic ability (the majority of practitioners have an incredibly powerful and toned body), the real benefits and purpose of yoga relate to what you can't see. They stress that handstands and fancy transitions have little to do with actual yoga. The purpose of building a stronger body is to support the deeper spiritual practices and build more compassion for yourself and others, to become a kinder, more caring person, and ultimately to increase *prana*.

VINYASA OR FLOW CLASSES

If you're interested in the Ashtanga yoga method but perhaps are looking for something a little less rigid with a little more creative sequencing, check out *vinyasa* or flow classes. The styles incorporate many of the same elements as those in Ashtanga yoga, with the exception of set series and some of the more traditional aspects of the Ashtanga yoga system.

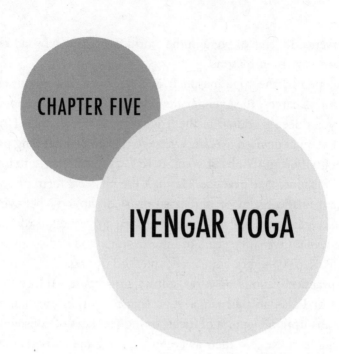

CHAPTER FIVE

IYENGAR YOGA

Health is a state of complete harmony of the body, mind, and spirit. When one is free from physical disabilities and mental distractions, the gates of the soul open.

— **B. K. S. IYENGAR,** founder of Iyengar yoga

Introduction: Spiritual Yoga in a Physical Form

Characterized by precision, Iyengar yoga is a highly disciplined practice that uses the physical experience of the body to develop consciousness. Students pay close attention to the anatomical details of each posture — the specific placement and spatial relationship of the hands and feet, torso, legs and arms, hips, shoulders, neck, and head — spreading awareness to every part of the body. A true mind-body discipline, the method systematically cultivates strength, flexibility, endurance, and stability along with correct structural alignment and concentration. It is one of the most widely practiced forms of yoga in the world, attracting a broad range of people for a variety of reasons.

Developed by the yoga master B. K. S. Iyengar throughout his long and illustrious career, the Iyengar method is an innovative approach to classical yoga deeply rooted in the Yoga Sutras of Patanjali. However, whereas Patanjali devised ashtanga yoga to depict an ascending progression through the eight limbs of yoga, B. K. S. Iyengar sought to integrate all eight limbs into one practice. He took the physical form of yoga and pushed it into the realm of higher spiritual disciplines, believing students could learn to meditate and refine their awareness through *asana* and *pranayama*. Over fifty years of intense study and dedicated personal practice, B. K. S. Iyengar engineered a method of yoga that, through the physical practice of yoga postures, allows students to explore the highest stages of Patanjali's ashtanga yoga (concentration, meditation, and complete absorption by point of focus, or higher states of consciousness). As students learn to hold their awareness in multiple individual parts of the body simultaneously, the concentration and sustained focus required to correctly align the yoga postures completely absorbs the mind in a meditative state, opening the gateway to higher states of consciousness. Iyengar yoga is thus considered a meditation in action.

PATANJALI'S ASHTANGA YOGA

Iyengar yoga uses *asana* and *pranayama* as the primary tools for refining awareness and mastering all eight stages of ashtanga yoga:

YAMA: Social discipline

NIYAMA: Personal discipline

ASANA: Yoga postures

PRANAYAMA: Breath control

PRATYAHARA: Sense withdrawal

DHARANA: Concentration

DHYANA: Meditation

SAMADHI: Complete absorption

In his classical treatise, Sage Patanjali maintains that yoga is for the stilling of the mind. However, if the body is in noticeable discomfort or pain,
it's nearly impossible for the mind to become quiet. The two are not separate but interconnected. When the body is ill, the mind also becomes lethargic and depressed; in order to still the mind, the body must be clear of pain.
In fact, your entire being is interrelated from the most physical layer down
to the essence of your innermost Self: What happens in one layer affects
every other layer. A complete approach to physical, mental, emotional, and
spiritual well-being, Iyengar yoga uses the physical experience of the body,
asana practice, to know the mind and penetrate the deeper aspects of Self.
The intensity and depth at which the method is physically practiced naturally bring about transformation on all levels of being.

A NEW APPROACH

Uniting the quests for physical well-being and spiritual transformation, B. K. S.
Iyengar created an accessible approach to classical yoga that allows the
everyday person to experience the wisdom of the Yoga Sutras.

The Gist: From the Known to the Unknown

The Iyengar method is a very individualized approach, making the style
of practice not only appropriate but also beneficial for all ages and abilities. Iyengar yoga is particularly suited for those with chronic conditions,
limitations, or special needs. B. K. S. Iyengar systematized over two hundred classical yoga postures, as well as fourteen types of *pranayama* (with
variations), ranging from basic to exceedingly advanced *asanas*, ensuring
that students gradually and safely progress through the syllabus of poses
as they develop strength, flexibility, balance, mind-body awareness, and
the ability to remain focused. Standing poses, which are heavily emphasized in beginning-level classes, are the foundation upon which the whole
Iyengar system of *asanas* is built. Dynamic and energizing, standing postures build strength and stability, improve coordination and circulation,
and increase general vitality. They are the easiest group of poses with

which to familiarize yourself with the major parts of your anatomical structure while learning correct body alignment from the feet up.

In your first few Iyengar yoga classes you will become oriented to the general shapes and basic elements of the beginning-level *asanas* (usually given by their Sanskrit names), which include mostly standing poses, some simple sitting poses, and basic inversions, as well as postures for deep relaxation. Slow to moderately paced, level 1 Iyengar yoga classes may have a start-stop feel to them, and you're likely to do the same pose multiple times in a row. Beginning with the foundation of a pose, the teacher will establish one key alignment point, such as pressing down the four corners of your feet in Tadasana (Standing Mountain Pose), and then have the students focus on the particular instruction when structuring the posture. Once that element of the pose is understood, the teacher will then introduce a second alignment point, building on the first. When the teacher dissects the various aspects of an *asana*, poses are organized methodically so that when you revisit one you'll be asked to apply the first alignment instruction, keep that action in place, and apply the next element of the posture as instructed. In that manner, the teacher will always guide students from what they've learned and now know, adding piece by piece what they yet need to know in order to perform the pose correctly and safely (going from the known to the unknown).

NEW TO THE IYENGAR METHOD

Whether you've been practicing yoga for years or are a complete novice, everyone new to the Iyengar system is asked to attend level 1 classes consistently for an extended period of time. Once you've developed a fundamental knowledge of the style's precise alignment and have integrated its basic principles, you will be introduced to the finer details of the postures in level 1/2 and level 2 classes. When you practice at the appropriate level and pace, the method systematically cultivates a complete understanding of the yoga *asanas*, starting with the basics and incorporating more intricate alignment details as your body and mind become capable of integrating the instructions.

The methodic nature in which the structure of the postures is organized often translates to long timings, that is, holding the pose for an extended period of time. Rather than moving quickly from one *asana* to the next, Iyengar yoga students take the necessary time to consciously move into the alignment of each pose and become stable, receiving benefits they may have otherwise missed. Iyengar yoga includes very little *vinyasa* flow (at least in the beginning stages of practice), and you shouldn't expect an intense cardiovascular workout. Nor should you expect to hear music during class. You should expect a highly developed teaching methodology, precise use of language, and clear demonstrations of how to achieve correct anatomical alignment in a posture. In Iyengar yoga, the emphasis is on learning (not just doing), and unlike in more experiential approaches that encourage students to explore their body in the yoga postures, there's definitely a right way to do the *asanas* in Iyengar yoga. Trained to look and see their students (never practicing along), teachers actively correct misalignment, giving individual feedback and manual physical adjustments as needed. Iyengar teachers are very skilled at offering posture modifications for simple injuries, such as low back or simple knee pain. In return, students are required to focus intently on what they're being asked to do in each pose.

When you visit an Iyengar yoga studio, one of the first things you'll notice is the large number of yoga props (straps, blocks, blankets, bolsters, chairs, ropes, etc.) around the classroom. The style is known for using props to facilitate learning and to help a variety of students create optimal body alignment and perform a posture correctly, minimizing the risk of strain or injury and allowing students of all ages and abilities to receive the full benefits of the *asanas*. B. K. S. Iyengar himself pioneered the use of yoga props, which have become commonplace in most yoga studios, adapting the *asanas* for a variety of physical limitations and conditions. In class, Iyengar yoga teachers will use props to modify the poses according to individual needs, allowing each student to practice within his or her healthy range of motion. Props also provide support as students hold a pose for a considerable amount of time, helping them find the balance between effort and relaxation and breathe more freely. Once a student is able to do a posture correctly, effectively, and with ease and stability, props are no longer used.

PRACTICING WITH PROPS

After laying down your yoga mat, grab two blankets, two blocks, and a strap, which you will use at the instruction of the teacher. If more props are needed he or she will let the students know when the time comes. Remember, Iyengar yoga is very specific and potentially very different from the alignment you may have previously practiced. Even if you don't think you need props, it's in your best interest to follow the teacher's instructions, using props regardless of how well you can already perform a pose. Teachers will often use props to emphasize a key action in the body you may not feel without their use.

Iyengar yoga *is* truly for everyone. The style of practice can be adapted to meet the needs of just about anyone who is interested in learning how to do yoga postures in alignment. However, despite the misconception, not all Iyengar yoga classes involve holding a handful of postures for long durations of time. Within the methodology, teachers have a fair amount of discretion, and classes can take on many diverse forms of practice, offering a wide variety of experiences once you've learned the fundamentals. During a particular class you could be asked to hold the poses, stopping in between to break down the posture's various elements, but, in the next, perform poses rapidly back-to-back with few or no demonstrations. The style also promotes a variety of postures, with an emphasis on inversions, particularly Supported Headstand (Salamba Sirsasana) and Shoulder Stand (Salamba Sarvangasana) for their profound therapeutic effects.

Almost all Iyengar yoga classes begin with a chant to honor Sage Patanjali, which is usually sung in a call-and-response manner and led by the teacher. Most studios provide printed cards of the invocation's Sanskrit transliteration for you to follow along. During class, more experienced Iyengar teachers will integrate yoga philosophy within the *asana* practice, imparting the wisdom of the Yoga Sutras to their students and discussing the relevance of the incorporation of practice into their daily lives. Class always ends with deep relaxation in Savasana, or Corpse Pose, which is a crucial aspect of the Iyengar method.

INVOCATION TO SAGE PATANJALI

Yogana cittasya padena vacam
malam sarirasya ca vaidyakena
yopakarottam paravaram muninam
patanjalinm pranajalirantao'smi
abahu purusakaram
sankha cakrasi dharinam
sahasra sirasan svetam
pranamami patanjalim

Let us bow before the noblest of sages Patanjali, who gave yoga for serenity and sanctity of mind, grammar for clarity and purity of speech and medicine for perfection of health. Let us prostrate before Patanjali, an incarnation of Adisesa, whose upper body has a human form, whose arms hold a conch and a disc, and who is crowned by a thousand-headed cobra.

Iyengar Alignment: The Practice of Precision

Using yoga *asana* to bring about transformative states of the mind, the Iyengar method gives primacy to the physical alignment of the body. Correct, or optimal, alignment is the precise position and spatial relationship of the bones in a posture, a precision that allows for equal amounts of stability and freedom in order to receive the maximum benefits of practice while also protecting the joints, ligaments, muscle fibers, and tendons — leaving little room for injury. When you exercise improperly, reinforcing misalignments, the tendency is to rely on the more-developed muscles for strength purposes and to continue to stretch (possibly overstretch or strain) the more flexible areas of the body. Practicing yoga *asana* in alignment encourages the tighter areas of the body to open and the weaker parts to strengthen, balancing and developing the body harmoniously.

Once the various bones are optimally aligned, less muscular effort is required, and the body can naturally relax in a pose, allowing the posture's beneficial effects to penetrate deeper.

PRACTICING CORRECT ALIGNMENT

Many students find that as their alignment improves, the yoga poses become less difficult, and also that aches, pains, and even stubborn musculoskeletal problems begin to dissolve. B. K. S. Iyengar is renowned worldwide for his extensive knowledge and application of yoga for therapeutic purposes, which is largely incorporated into the style's teaching methodology. When you attend Iyengar yoga classes you will learn how to use the practice to diminish discomforts, ease minor ailments, and relieve stress.

Iyengar alignment is exacting and requires that rigorous attention be paid in an *asana*. Working with deliberate purpose, you will begin to bring your awareness to individual parts of your body in order to move into the proper alignment of the poses, establishing a continual mind-body connection. Once such awareness has been cultivated, movement is no longer aimless but very precise and intentional. The Iyengar method emphasizes the distinction between intelligent action and random movement: the difference between throwing your hands up in the air without thinking about what you're doing (random movement) and engaging specific muscles to initiate the action of lifting your hands overhead with concentrated effort (intelligent action). The first is often a result of momentum, whereas the latter is a product of aligned integration (in this case, integration of the arm bones, shoulders, and upper body to raise your hands). B. K. S. Iyengar has said that without awareness there is no intelligence, and the final pose is achieved only when the body is aligned and infused with both.

Beyond the placement of the bones, Iyengar alignment addresses the organic, or physiological, body as well. The way in which you practice yoga, how you do specific poses, greatly affects your internal organs and their associated systems, such as the cardiovascular, respiratory, reproductive, endocrine, and nervous systems. Organs in general secrete a variety of hormones and other chemicals; the amount of chemicals released into your system and the timing of their release can fluctuate according to the way you move and align your body. Different yoga postures push on specific organs and glands, disturbing their natural rhythms and creating various physiological effects. When the body is out of alignment, certain organs are not in their correct anatomical position and pressing on them creates an undesirable effect, such as a sudden increase in emotional or hormonal levels. For example, twisting poses squeeze the pelvic and abdominal organs, massaging and toning the stomach, gastrointestinal tract, gall bladder, liver, kidneys, and spleen. Once the twist is released, new blood floods into the region, improving circulation and flushing out toxins from the various organs. However, if you twist unconsciously or overdo a twist, you may experience a sudden surge of anger or become grumpy and irritated from the overproduction of bile by the liver. Meanwhile, overdoing backbends elicits a different hormonal-emotional response, and really overdoing backbends while menstruating can cause a woman to lose her period for a length of time. Therefore, trained Iyengar yoga teachers are required to have a deep-seated knowledge of the body and yoga *asanas*, always taking the physiological and emotional effects of each pose into consideration. Furthermore, a balanced sequence will tone not only the muscles, ligaments, and other soft tissues of the musculoskeletal system but also the organs, glands, and nerves of the body.

However, Iyengar alignment doesn't end there: The rigorous practice has as much to do with the subtle, or energetic, body as it does with the actual physical body — helping to refine all layers of your being from the physical to the mental to the emotional to the energetic and spiritual. In paying close attention to the biomechanical alignment of the yoga *asanas*, the method also focuses on the subtle internal movements of energy (*prana*) throughout the body. According to the yoga tradition, *prana* permeates all facets of our being: physical, mental, emotional, sexual, and spiritual. When your physical body is out of alignment, you incur blockages within your energetic body, impeding the flow of *prana* and creating dis-ease. As you practice yoga postures in correct anatomical alignment, blockages are dissolved, allowing the optimal flow of *prana* through the body. You can also build energy in one region of your body by bringing your awareness to that area, working in a specific way, and guiding *prana* through the breath to promote healing.

MORE THAN WHAT MEETS THE EYE

Although Iyengar yoga emphasizes the physical practice of *asanas*, the method is about so much more than developing strength, flexibility, and correct anatomical alignment. It also involves work on all layers of being and their interconnectedness. Regular and disciplined practice will improve your physiological health, emotional stability, and spiritual well-being, as well as increase mental clarity and receptivity.

Class Orchestration: Sequencing

There are three key elements that distinguish Iyengar yoga from other forms of yoga practice: technique (precise anatomical alignment), timing (long holds), and intelligent sequencing. The order in which certain yoga *asanas* are done has a powerful cumulative effect and is therefore taken very seriously in the Iyengar method. In general, poses are sequenced in a manner that develops strength, flexibility, balance, and stamina, as well as skill and understanding of body alignment from posture to posture and class to class. Beyond that, the combination of *asanas* and the specific order in which they are performed intensifies the emotional, mental, and energetic effects of practice, essentially transforming all layers of being.

Following certain principles and general guidelines within the method, teachers are encouraged to use their creativity when designing sequences. One of the first things taken into consideration is the level and condition of the students in class, followed by the time of day, the time of year, what the weather is like, what's going on in the world, and so forth. From there, teachers will determine what the focus for class is going to be. On different days, teachers promote different aspects of the practice, whether it's building strength, increasing flexibility, integrating those two, or something else entirely. The focus could be on standing poses, balancing poses, inversions, forward folds, or backbends; it could be on restorative postures and deep relaxation or on *pranayama* and increasing the circulation of energy through the body. Additionally, there are sequences (and entire programs) for specific conditions and ailments, such as menstruation, pregnancy, menopause, headaches, insomnia, depression, arthritis, high blood pressure, immunodeficiency, and more. B. K. S. Iyengar designed many of these at the Ramamani Iyengar Memorial Yoga Institute, in Pune, India, where after nearly seventy years of teaching, he continues to refine his method with his daughter Geeta S. Iyengar and his son Prashant S. Iyengar.

SYMPHONY OF *ASANAS*

Teachers will often link the yoga poses in such a way that each *asana* is preparation for the next, more difficult posture, building the poses sequentially upon one another. Beginning with standing poses and ending with quieter, more introspective postures, sequences are designed to create a culminating effect (similar to a symphony or drama) with a continuous mounting toward one or two more exhilarating and challenging *asanas* followed by a coming down or mellowing before complete relaxation in Savasana.

The Next Stage of Practice: *Pranayama*

The practice of *pranayama* (breath control techniques) is considered separate from the development of breath awareness and deep breathing in the Iyengar method. Every class involves conscious breathing; however, Iyengar students aren't introduced to *pranayama* practices until they've demonstrated a firm foundation in their *asana* practice. Considered an advanced discipline, *pranayama* can have serious effects on the central nervous system of the body, which can be felt almost immediately, so should be practiced under the guidance of an experienced teacher (as stressed by B. K. S. Iyengar). Students are introduced to basic *pranayama* techniques only after they have practiced *asana* for at least three months, building the strength, flexibility, and correct alignment necessary to sit upright with an open chest for certain lengths of time. Plus, after observing a student's *asana* practice for a few months, the teacher will be able to determine if his or her nervous system is steady enough for *pranayama* practices, which can be very destabilizing and cause someone to become anxious or angry, even seriously ill in worst-case scenarios.

However, if practiced correctly, a steady *pranayama* practice has numerous beneficial effects. *Pranayama* will not only increase the circulation of *pranic* energy through the body — increasing physical vitality — but also tone the circulatory, nervous, respiratory, and digestive systems, as well as activate and invigorate the various internal organs. What's more, *pranayama* is an essential precursor to seated meditation. Controlling the breath through *pranayama* brings the mind and senses under control, taking you very deep into yourself and preparing you for the experience of meditation. When the breath becomes steady and smooth, the mind becomes still, and the process of withdrawing the senses can begin. A peaceful inner presence is cultivated, leading to the inner state of meditation.

NEW TO *PRANAYAMA?*

Pranayama is traditionally taught in a seated, cross-legged position, or Lotus Pose; however, B. K. S. Iyengar recommends that students practicing *pranayama* for the first time start in a supine position. He also cautions that if at any time you experience tension or pain in your head while performing *pranayama* exercises, you should release the breathing technique and allow the breath to return to normal.

Above the Rest: Teaching Credentials

After its primary distinction — precise alignment and rigorous attention to detail — the Iyengar style of yoga distinguishes itself secondarily with the competency and accreditation of its instructors. Combine the two — highly trained instructors teaching correct physical alignment — and the method is one of the safest, most effective forms of yoga to practice. Certification as an Iyengar yoga instructor ensures that the teacher has a certain knowledge of the body, anatomically, physiologically, and energetically, and a profound understanding of the yoga *asanas*, as well as the knowledge of how to modify and use the postures therapeutically to heal common ailments and address injuries.

The certification process for becoming an Iyengar yoga teacher is one of the most thorough and demanding in the yoga world. A student must first demonstrate a strong commitment to the Iyengar system, attending three classes a week as well as maintaining a daily home practice, for a minimum of three years before becoming eligible to apply for and attend a sanctioned Iyengar yoga teacher training. He or she must also have developed a close relationship with a certified teacher who agrees to mentor him or her through the long certification process. It takes at least two years of rigorous training, including an apprenticeship, to become certified at the introductory level. The teacher-in-training must also pass two standardized assessments, including written exams on anatomy, yoga philosophy, and practical knowledge of teaching, in addition to undergoing careful observation and a strict evaluation of his or her personal *asana* and *pranayama* practices and ability to teach a class of students. Once all of these assessments are completed and approved, the trainee is considered an introductory II instructor and is legally permitted to use the trademarked Iyengar yoga name commercially as long as he or she remains committed to achieving the purity, excellence, and high standards of the system.

HIGH EXPECTATIONS

Certified Iyengar yoga teachers are expected to maintain a regular personal practice, continue to train with a senior teacher or by traveling to the Iyengar institute in India, and earnestly teach the Iyengar method without incorporating other styles of yoga or disciplines. They are also expected to uphold the ethical guidelines provided by the board of directors of the Iyengar Yoga National Association of the United States.

The majority of teachers go on to spend years, even a decade or more, training at the subsequent intermediate and advanced levels, completing increasingly difficult assessment processes with higher standards and new material along the way. Beyond the minimum certification required to teach Iyengar yoga, which takes a bare minimum of five years to achieve, there are six intermediate levels (junior intermediate I, II, and III and senior intermediate I, II, and III) and six advanced levels (junior advanced I, II, and III and senior advanced I, II, and III) of certification. Once a teacher starts training at the junior intermediate II level, he or she is required to study at least once at the Ramamani Iyengar Memorial Yoga Institute, in Pune, India, and beginning at the senior intermediate II level, certification must be granted by B.K.S. Iyengar himself. Aside from increasing levels of competency in the art and science of teaching yoga, advanced training and additional certifications allow Iyengar yoga teachers to work with special-needs populations, such as students with multiple sclerosis, and to apply the various therapeutic aspects of the *asana* practice to a multitude of conditions and limitations.

IYENGAR YOGA TEACHERS

You will find a variety of teaching personalities and attitudes within the Iyengar yoga system. Some teachers are very serious in approaching the methodology, and some are more lighthearted; some are forceful and sometimes harsh (like B.K.S. Iyengar himself), and others are gentler and more sensitive; some like to go slow, and others like to go fast. Given the method's strong foundation and rigorous requirements, teachers have many opportunities to express themselves.

Conclusion

Iyengar yoga is the perfect place to start if you are new to the practice. The knowledge of alignment gained in the Iyengar method will serve you in any style of yoga you choose to go on to study, and the self-awareness and concentration gained will benefit you in all areas of your life. Even if you've been practicing yoga for years, dropping in on a few beginner Iyengar classes will give you a whole new understanding of the *asanas* and add another layer of depth to your practice. Many students arrive at the method searching for more in their yoga classes, whether it's the individual attention, detailed alignment, or mental focus, and end up staying for a lifetime. What's more, after years, even decades, of practice, they aren't bored yet, but the style does tend to attract those with a curious mind, and the complexity and subtlety of the system present endless opportunities for exploration.

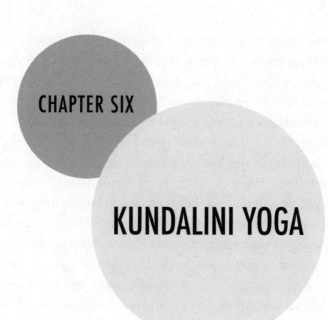

CHAPTER SIX

KUNDALINI YOGA

Kundalini yoga classes are a dynamic blend of postures, *pranayama*, *mantra*, music and meditation, which teach you the art of relaxation, self-healing and elevation. Balancing body and mind enables you to experience the clarity and beauty of your soul.

— **YOGI BHAJAN, PhD**, founder of Kundalini yoga

Introduction: The Yoga of Experience

Kundalini yoga as taught by Yogi Bhajan is a highly spiritual and dynamic practice aimed at expanding consciousness and increasing physical vitality by accessing and integrating subtle life-force energy throughout the body. Less concerned with how this style of yoga looks, Kundalini yoga emphasizes the effects of its practice and the principle that "experiencing is believing." The style is about direct, personal experience and awareness. Using movement, rhythm, breath, and sound, the practice effectively stimulates and shifts your energy — something you can actually *feel* in your body. That energy is your essence. The science of Kundalini yoga was developed to give you a direct experience of your soul, connecting you to your highest consciousness and divine identity within, so that you can realize your highest potential and fulfill your personal destiny.

Kept in secret for thousands of years, *kundalini* yoga was verbally passed from master to disciple until 1969, when Yogi Bhajan decided to openly teach the ancient technology in the States. *Why?* Compassion. He desired an end to suffering. He believed that all human beings deserve to be healthy, happy, and whole and that the powerful technology should be made available to everyone, that in fact modern society needs Kundalini yoga to be able to handle the difficult challenges of our time. He recognized the unlimited potential for spiritual growth and fulfillment within every individual and aspired to help people connect with their innate beauty and power to excel in this lifetime. A *kundalini* yoga master at the age of sixteen, Yogi Bhajan had access to a legacy of techniques and spiritual wisdom, which he bestowed to his students and teachers over a period of thirty-five years. Though he attracted hundreds of followers, Bhajan always affirmed that it was never his intention to gain disciples; instead, he sought to train teachers with a method for healing, uplifting, and inspiring humanity. In 1972 he founded the Kundalini Research Institute, later structuring an international teaching certification comprising three levels. Today there are thousands of Kundalini yoga teachers worldwide.

THE AQUARIAN AGE

Yogi Bhajan was concerned with preparing people for the radical shift from the Pisces age to the Aquarian age, which he predicted to be complete on November 11, 2011. Ruled by awareness, this new age marks a transition into higher consciousness. The frequency of the planet's energy is believed to be more intense than ever before. Yogi Bhajan believed that a person's greatest tool for navigating such a powerful change is his or her intuition and connection to the divine source within.

Beyond the science and technology of Kundalini yoga, Yogi Bhajan taught his students how to live according to own their intuition, how to consciously structure their lives, how to communicate and have relationships, and how to be of service. He even imparted lessons on how to attract prosperity and live an abundant, joyful life. The beloved leader promoted a yogic lifestyle, and his teachings covered a wide array of topics, including hygiene, nutrition, marriage, child rearing, female empowerment, numerology, compassion, and much more. Shortly after arriving in the States, Yogi Bhajan founded the 3HO (Healthy, Happy, Holy Organization) Foundation, which continues to serve as a "Global Community of Living Yoga" for those who are immersed in the Kundalini yoga lifestyle and practice the master's teachings on a daily basis.

KUNDALINI YOGA AS TAUGHT BY YOGI BHAJAN

There are many different branches, or lineages, within the larger *kundalini yoga* tradition. This chapter focuses on the highly structured and widely practiced system Kundalini yoga, which intersects with the Sikh lineage of masters. Bhajan himself was a devoted Sikh given the first-ever title of "Siri Singh Sahib," with the responsibility of establishing Sikh *Dharma* in the West. Though many of his followers also took up Sikhism, Bhajan never pushed his religion on his students. Kundalini yoga is not a Sikh religious practice and is open to all faiths.

The Kundalini yoga tradition is, and always has been, a system for householders, meaning that the technology was designed for those who choose not to withdraw from the world in search of spiritual attainment. Originally, classical yoga (the yoga of Patanjali's Yoga Sutras) was intended for renunciants and ascetics who turned away from everyday life, steering clear of the entrapments of incarnate life in pursuit of radical autonomy and Self-realization. As society's outcasts, these holy men, unshaven, filthy, and barely clothed, lived in remote caves and forests, where they could dedicate themselves entirely to their spiritual endeavors. In contrast, Kundalini yoga involves a *tantric* path meant for those who have homes and families, jobs and worldly responsibilities, and who seek to balance their inner and outer worlds.

Because Kundalini yoga is for those with demanding worldly lives, time is of the essence. The system was scientifically developed to efficiently and effectively create the desired changes in yourself and your life more quickly than is possible with other styles of yoga (prompting a resounding affirmation among Kundalini yoga teachers and practitioners). Whether it's to reduce anxiety, lose weight, be healthier and happier, live with more passion, or gain clarity and so forth, change is the primary motivation for practicing. Kundalini yoga claims to be particularly effective because the method systematically affects all aspects of your being — mental, emotional, physical, and spiritual — to create permanent change in your life. In fact, Kundalini yoga guarantees change. If you're not interested in a shift, then this practice may not be for you. Yogi Bhajan often said, "Kundalini yoga is for everyone, but not everyone is ready for it."

The Gist: Class Journey

Kundalini yoga is multidimensional, involving yogic exercises, breathing techniques, meditations, hand gestures (*mudras*), and chanting. It is perhaps the most comprehensive class experience among styles of yoga and is certainly more dynamic than the static array of postures presented in a traditional *hatha* yoga class. The practice alternates between active exercises and periods of relaxation, during which you'll be guided to pay close attention to any internal sensations that may be taking place. There's a definite inner focus to Kundalini yoga practice, and you'll be reminded throughout class to keep your attention focused inwardly. The goal is not to perfect poses but to cultivate greater levels of awareness in order to have a deeper experience of yourself.

After tuning in with the Adi Mantra, practice begins with a short *pranayama* exercise followed by five to ten minutes of warm-ups to prepare the body before settling into the main work of the class. Warm-ups generally include movements such as cat-cow, body and neck rolls, Sun Salutations, moving bridges, and so forth. If you've practiced other styles of yoga before coming to Kundalini, you'll most likely be familiar with the poses performed in the beginning of class. Once the body and spine are warm and more flexible, the teacher will guide you into your first *kriya*, a yogic exercise specific to Kundalini yoga, followed by a minirelaxation and tuning in, then on to the next exercise. A longer relaxation in the form of Savasana (Corpse Pose) is held for five to fifteen minutes at the conclusion of practice prior to seated meditation. All Kundalini yoga classes are formatted in a similar order, closing with the blessing song, "May the Long Time Sun Shine upon You."

In general, the class environment is warm, friendly, and supportive. Props and modifications are gladly given to those who aren't comfortable in a position or with a movement, so if you are experiencing any pain (particularly in the knees, considering many exercises are performed in a seated or kneeling position), please let the teacher know; he or she will be more than happy to help. The style is beginner-friendly and very doable. You don't have to be in tip-top shape or be superflexible to practice Kundalini yoga. All you need is to be able to breathe and move, and you will have an energetic experience in your very first class. You may even achieve results, such as relief from stress or insomnia, right off the bat. By moving and activating all parts of the body, Kundalini yoga strengthens the nervous and immune systems, improves circulation, and stimulates gland secretion so that every system of the body functions optimally and physical health is restored. Ultimately, the practice is meant to heal, relax, and simultaneously recharge your entire being.

WHY THE WHITE?

You will immediately notice that almost all Kundalini yoga teachers and students wear white and wrap their head with a scarf or turban. They do so to expand their aura and contain the energy in the higher brain centers, respectively. Wearing white, wrapping your head, and not cutting your hair are aspects of the 3HO lifestyle, which is more prevalent in Kundalini yoga centers than in mixed-style studios. Either place, you aren't expected to wear white, but you are encouraged to wear loose, comfortable clothing and natural fibers.

Well beyond mere physical exercise, Kundalini yoga is designed to work on the subtle body to bring about profound energetic effects aimed at elevating your consciousness and promoting feelings of connection, peace, and oneness. It's definitely one of the most palpably spiritual class environments among yoga styles, but you don't have to believe in anything in particular. Kundalini yoga is about connecting with yourself on a deeper level; what you call that connection (divinity, God, cosmic consciousness, Buddha, nature) is up to you. Remember, you are there to have an experience of your highest Self in your body, that's all. However, all the exercises, techniques, and terms can be a bit overwhelming. Try not to get caught up in the language or science of things. Don't worry if everything doesn't make sense at first; you'll grasp more over time, and the style's mystery is part of its mystique and allure. The teacher is there to guide you. Nothing is expected of you, except that you come with an open mind and try your best.

Kundalini Energy: The Sleeping Serpent

The exact science of Kundalini yoga (referring to specific meditation techniques that generate specific effects or outcomes) was developed as a direct and efficient means to access and integrate *kundalini-shakti*, the primordial power of the universe embodied in every individual. Like *prana*, this power is a basic bioenergy; however, *kundalini* is a much more powerful and potent force that remains dormant in most people, while *prana* is active, is more accessible, and can be sensed more readily in the body. Not to be underestimated, *prana* maintains the functions of the body and mind, keeping your entire system in working order. Without *prana* there would be no life. On the other hand, *kundalini-shakti* is the cosmic energy of consciousness that propels psychospiritual growth and healing in all human beings. It's a wellspring of creative energy, the boundless energy of your soul representing your immense capacity and power to thrive.

Kundalini energy dwells in a potential state at the base of the spine, ready and waiting to be released. Once activated, the vibration of *kundalini* initiates a process of spiritual development that leads to the realization of your true nature and mergence with universal consciousness. The cosmic energy increases spiritual capacity when awakened in an individual. As psychic energy, *kundalini* moves through the subtle body, breaking apart stuck patterns in your cellular makeup and psyche — deconstructing your personal identity, which has sustained the experience of separation. The energy is drawn up along the spine to activate the higher centers of the brain, opening you to deeper levels of sensitivity and receptivity and broadening your perspective beyond the normal capacities of the conditioned mind. Your entire consciousness expands, so much so that you begin to sense that everything and everyone is part of you. Accessing your brain's higher centers increases your mind's capacity to first imagine and then experience your infinite Self beyond limited notions of reality. The heightened state is usually temporary (you inevitably return to your normal orientation); however, the shift in perspective is not completely lost, and with more sensitivity and awareness than before, you begin to live your life from an elevated place.

A TRANSFORMATIONAL PRACTICE

By clearing the way for *kundalini* energy to move freely through the body, the practice of Kundalini yoga releases old tensions and emotional and mental patterns that keep you removed from your center of truth, inner clarity, and innate wisdom. More and more aspects of your soul are revealed as you establish an inner connection with your true Self, as though you were removing dust from the mirror of your heart.

Often depicted as a sleeping serpent, *kundalini-shakti* is said to be coiled three and a half turns around the sacrum (the Romans called the bone *os sacrum* after the Greek heroine Osteon, meaning "sacred bone") in the root *chakra*. Awakened, *kundalini* ascends through the body's central energy channel, known as the *shushmana*, until it culminates in the crown *chakra* at the top of the skull. Simply defined, *chakras* are focal points of pooled energy within the concept of the subtle body. Seven main *chakras* are associated with *kundalini* rising, each corresponding to a position in the physical body and responsible for specific functions in various dimensions of being. They relate to different aspects of our human nature, influencing everything from our mood and thoughts to our physical health and behavior, as well as our personal and spiritual development. The three lower energy centers deal with our basic biological needs, and the higher *chakras* correspond to the spiritual realms. Kundalini yoga was designed to balance and coordinate the functions of the first three *chakras*, allowing *kundalini* energy to flow up the spine to awaken awareness in the upper *chakras*, giving you an experience of your highest consciousness.

THE EIGHTH *CHAKRA*

Your aura, the electromagnetic field encircling your physical body, is also considered a *chakra* in the Kundalini yoga tradition, for a total of eight *chakras* rather than the traditional seven. The eighth *chakra* represents radiance and protection, combining and integrating the effects of all the *chakras*. When all seven main *chakras* are balanced, your aura fully radiates and you feel vibrant, healthy, and more expansive.

In Sanskrit, the word *chakra* literally means "wheel" or "circle," and *chakras* are generally thought of as spinning disks of energy. When open and operating optimally, they radiate *prana* through their region of the body via hundreds of subtle energy tubes called *nadis* (according to ancient yogic texts, the subtle body contains seventy-two thousand *nadis*); however, the centers are often knotted, restricting the circulation of energy. Blocked or weak *chakras* create imbalances associated with problematic effects, such as lethargy, insecurity, and addictions, even physical pain and sickness. For example, when someone is experiencing a blockage in her throat *chakra*, it isn't uncommon for that person to have neck and shoulder pain or even tonsillitis. She may also have difficulty speaking up for herself. A blockage in the root *chakra* often manifests as low back pain, digestive problems, and lack of energy and is associated with feelings of being overwhelmed by life that can lead to anxiety and depression. On the other hand, when the *chakras* are activated and the flow of energy between the centers is harmonized, we experience a greater sense of self and peace, more clarity and connection, and good health.

THE *CHAKRAS*

First, or root, *chakra*: Muladhara *Chakra* (red)
>   Located at the end of the tailbone; governs the organs and functions of elimination. Associated with foundation, security, survival, stability, courage, and self-acceptance.

Second, or sacral, *chakra*: Svadisthana *Chakra* (orange)
>   Located at the sacrum and sex organs; governs the sexual organs and reproductive system. Associated with creativity, desire, sensuality, sexuality, adaptability, and emotional identity.

Third, or navel, *chakra*: Manipura *Chakra* (yellow)
>   Located just above the navel point at the solar plexus; governs the digestive and autonomic nervous systems. Associated with willpower, commitment, confidence, mental agility, autonomy, and personality.

Fourth, or heart, *chakra*: Anahata *Chakra* (green)
>   Located at the center of the chest; governs the heart, lungs, and thymus gland, as well as the circulation of energy throughout the body. Associated with love, compassion, humanity, openness, forgiveness, and peace.

Fifth, or throat, *chakra*: Visuddha *Chakra* (blue)
>   Located at the throat; governs the thyroid gland and speech organs, as well as communication. Associated with communication, sound vibration, ability to hear and speak the truth, creative identity, and intelligence.

Sixth, or forehead, *chakra*: Ajna *Chakra* (indigo)
>   Located between the eyebrows; governs the brain and pituitary gland. Associated with intuition, wisdom, awareness, imagination, vision, power of perception that transcends duality, and realization.

Seventh, or crown, *chakra*: Sahasrara *Chakra* (violet)
>   Located at the top of the head; governs the cerebrum and pineal gland. Associated with spirituality, transcendence, cosmic connection, pure awareness, god-consciousness, humility, and vastness.

The practice of Kundalini yoga is geared toward opening the *chakras* and purifying the energy channels, so that once its path is free, *kundalini-shakti* can gently and naturally be set in motion up the spine without force. As *kundalini* ascends the *shushmana*, it works to further release various contractions in the subtle body, activating, balancing, and connecting all seven *chakras* in turn along the way. The upward movement of *kundalini* through the *chakras* is typically gradual; it can even take years of genuine spiritual practice for *kundalini* to rise (though there are accounts of it spontaneously rising). Once the cosmic energy reaches the crown *chakra*, activating the dormant potential of the brain, complete spiritual unfoldment is said to occur. Here, the animated human life force binds with universal, or cosmic, consciousness in the merging of individual self and God.

IS KUNDALINI DANGEROUS?

Spontaneous *kundalini* awakening is associated with some serious side effects and can be dangerous for someone who has never practiced Kundalini yoga, which prepares the body for the surge of energy. When *kundalini* is stimulated through the primarily mental practices of meditation and visualization without physical preparation, the body has a difficult time handling the higher frequencies associated with the cosmic energy. Kundalini yoga, on the other hand, strengthens the nervous system, systematically trains the psyche, and aligns the body to hold the powerful vibrations of *kundalini-shakti*.

Chakras work through their physical counterparts, the endocrine glands. Human consciousness is in part biochemical in nature, which is to say that the chemicals secreted in the brain directly affect your consciousness and how you experience yourself and the world at large. Your emotions are a product of the biochemical processes in your brain. Hormones, such as endorphins, instantly affect the way you feel emotionally, even physically, which, in turn, influences your state of mind and perception of your immediate experience. Changes in your biochemistry change the way you feel and think, including your perception of reality.

When *kundalini-shakti* rises to the crown *chakra*, the energy activates the pituitary and pineal glands, causing them to secrete certain chemicals in the brain — altering your state of consciousness. (Yogi Bhajan initially introduced the practice of Kundalini yoga to a generation of youth experimenting with psychedelics to achieve the same effect.)

While the functions of the pineal gland remained a mystery to Western science until the twentieth century, mystical and yogic traditions have understood its important role in spiritual awakening for centuries. Related to divine thought, the pineal gland, located near the center of the brain, is considered the highest and most powerful source of ethereal energy available to humans. The pea-sized gland is known as the "seat of consciousness" and is linked to psychic development and intuition. The pituitary gland, on the other hand, is known as "the seat of the mind," representing the individual self, its two lobes (anterior and posterior) associated with regulating emotional thoughts and comprehending intellectual concepts. When both glands are stimulated, as they are in the practice of Kundalini yoga, their vibrations unite to activate the third-eye center, opening the doorway to higher consciousness.

THE INNER MIND'S EYE

Sometimes referred to as the sixth sense, the third-eye center is the gateway to the inner realms of consciousness, which cannot be perceived by the direct senses and normal faculties of the mind but rather are intuitively felt and seen. Your ability to sense subtle energies, as well as greater dimensions of reality, resides in your third eye. When you open and expand your third-eye center, your intuition flows freely, and the mind is flooded with infinite wisdom, insight, and inspiration.

Western science now knows that the pineal gland is involved in the secretion of melatonin, an important hormone that regulates the body's internal clock and circadian rhythms, such as sleep cycles, and that the pituitary gland releases endorphins, reducing levels of cortisol (a damaging stress hormone). The pituitary also manages the entire body's balance of hormones and their functions, such as sexual development, body temperature, and thyroid activity, acting as a command center that communicates with all the lower endocrine glands. Many Kundalini yoga exercises are designed to stimulate the pituitary, which, in its frequent mentions in class, is sometimes referred to as the "master gland" and is governed by the sixth *chakra*. In fact, the locations of the seven main *chakras* along the spine are similar to the locations of the major glands in the endocrine system, as well as to the locations of the various nerve bundles of the central nervous system, called ganglions, which move up the spine. By using scientific techniques aimed at activating individual *chakras*, the practice of Kundalini yoga strengthens the nervous system and stimulates gland secretion, helping regulate all physiological systems of the body.

Kriyas: Awakening Kundalini

The initial awakening of *kundalini-shakti* is often associated with an intense or concentrated experience, such as a near-death incident, deep meditation, or spiritual practice that involves techniques to manipulate energy. Kundalini yoga is considered a particularly powerful method in this arena, because the exercises are multidimensional, using multiple techniques, *asana*, *pranayama*, *mantras*, *mudras*, and expressive movements simultaneously to stimulate *kundalini* rising. Overall the practice is designed to restore the body, open energy channels, and calm the mind — clearing the way for spirit (the energy of higher consciousness) to move spontaneously and freely through you.

In Kundalini yoga the short, simple sequences of coordinated movements, poses, breathing patterns, internal chanting, and body locks are known as *kriyas*. The word *kriya* means "action." Yogi Bhajan said, "It is an action which must sprout seed." Each *kriya*, either a single action or a synergistic series of movements, known as a set, is a complete process in itself, designed to create a specific energetic effect. Every exercise is scientifically structured and intended to have a predictable physiological, energetic, or psychospiritual outcome or a combination of any of these. There are hundreds of prescribed sets as given by Yogi Bhajan: *kriyas* to improve your immune system; to increase your metabolism; to detoxify your liver; to balance your pelvis; to strengthen your core; and to calm your mind, as well as sequences for good fortune; for working through creative blocks; for mastering your mood; for tapping your intuition; for igniting your internal flame; and so forth. By improving the basic functions and various systems of the body, *kriyas* consistently practiced initiate a process of change that allows for healing and personal growth to happen.

The sheer number of yogic exercises and meditation techniques and their varying effects allow Kundalini yoga teachers to choose *kriyas* and create each class for a specific intention, such as "to brighten your energy." Because the method works on your subtle body, a short lecture or talk is often given at the beginning of class to convey the intention and energetic journey you and your classmates are about to experience. Guided by the teacher, who will often explain not only how to perform a particular action but also the effects of the *kriya*, you will either hold one position while practicing a specific, often rapid, breathing technique or move rhythmically in a pose for a certain length of time determined by the teacher (usually for three, eleven, or twenty-two minutes). In either case, the exercises can be quite dynamic, and moving and breathing at a pace that's comfortable for you is imperative. Seemingly easy at first, even basic *kriyas* can feel increasingly challenging; within minutes you'll most likely start to feel a burning sensation or fatigue in the areas of your body that are working. Kundalini yoga teachers are very positive and will encourage you to stay with it — to stay with the breath, the exercise, the moment — and simply notice whatever comes up for you, especially any negative thoughts or personal judgments, with an attitude of acceptance.

Part of the transformational journey involves challenging yourself to push slightly beyond what you perceive your limits to be. By doing so, you train yourself not to adhere to the limitations of the ordinary mind, and you can begin to experience expanded states of being. However, one of the main goals of Kundalini yoga is to feel good in your body; therefore, physically straining is counterproductive to your practice. If you need to slow down, take breaks, or rest, you're encouraged to do so as well. As with anything else, the more you practice, the more adept you will become at completing the various *kriyas* while remaining comfortable.

INNER GAZE

Kundalini exercises and meditations are practiced with your eyes shut in order to keep energy contained inside. Unless otherwise specified, your inner *drishti* (gaze) should focus on the "third-eye point." Once your eyes are closed, gently turn them upward and inward toward the center of your forehead.

Depending on the set and exercises chosen, classes can range from calm and meditative to vigorous and challenging. Basic, or single-action, *kriyas* usually involve rhythmic movement between two positions in an *asana*, such as rotating your torso left to right in a simple seated position, rocking back and forth on your pelvis in Bow Pose, or raising and lowering your legs while lying on your back. *Kriya* sets are longer sequences than single-action *kriyas*, involving multiple exercises and poses. In class you'll most likely have the opportunity to practice a few single-action *kriyas* within a larger set, which tends to involve a lot of flip-flopping around. (First you're sitting, then standing, then lying, then kneeling, then sitting again — you never know!) You may even feel a bit silly at first, expressively moving and breathing in unfamiliar patterns, so come to class with an open mind and a willingness to simply experience the practice of Kundalini yoga. A sense of humor also helps. Deeply spiritual, classes are also lighthearted and fun. Laughter is not uncommon. One Kundalini yoga teacher said that while it may look weird to someone watching, the first impression of someone participating in class may be, "This is incredible. I have never felt this energized and alive." The issue then becomes whether you can get out of your own way and immerse yourself in the experience.

Power of the Breath

Every Kundalini yoga exercise is supported and enhanced by a prescribed way of breathing, whether it's taking long, deep breaths, inhaling/exhaling with every movement, or doing a specific *pranayama* technique. One of the fundamental understandings of the tradition is that *prana* (life force) is received with every breath. By manipulating the breath, slowing it down, speeding it up, holding it in, and so forth, not only can you access more *prana*, but you can also stimulate and direct the flow of energy within your body. Kundalini yoga teaches you how to cultivate and use the *pranic* energy received with the air as you inhale. One of the first breathing techniques you'll learn is commonly referred to as yogic, or conscious, breathing. Done in and out of the nostrils, yogic breathing is slow, long, and deep, breathing down into your lower abdomen. Consciously slowing and deepening the breath quiets the mind and begins to calm down the nervous system, allowing you to be more present while inducing a state of peace and relaxation. From the very beginning of class you'll be directed time and again to bring your awareness to your breath.

DEEP BREATH, CALM MIND

Kundalini yoga teaches that the breath and state of mind are intricately linked. Shallow, rapid breaths indicate a state of stress, and long, deep inhalations and exhalations (fewer than ten breaths per minute) can create a peaceful, calm state. Taking four or fewer breaths per minute induces a deeply meditative state.

Unlike most yoga classes that use an *ujjayi* breath consistently throughout the *asana* portion of practice, Kundalini yoga mixes it up, using various breathing techniques in one class. Many of the exercises involve rhythmic movements done at the rate of your breath — for example, inhaling and exhaling as you raise and lower your shoulders, tilt your pelvis forward and back, or move your arms in an orchestrated pattern. In general, it's better to start more slowly in order to establish a rhythm with your breath and movements and then pick up the pace as you get the hang of things. A number of *kriyas* also require you to hold one posture, such as a squat with your arms outstretched in front of your heart, and to use a more vigorous breath to quicken and intensify the desired effects. In such cases, "Breath of Fire" is typically the go-to technique.

A powerful *pranayama*, Breath of Fire is an extremely effective way to cleanse the energy channels and move *prana* through the *chakras*. The rapid-breathing technique charges the entire nervous system, causing glands to secrete, purifying the bloodstream and energizing the body and mind. It is often one of the first exercises in class and is used consistently throughout Kundalini yoga, so much so that a teacher might assume you know the technique so may not always explain it in full detail in every class. The Breath of Fire is a continuous breath powered by abdominal contractions on the exhalation as the air is rhythmically pushed out and pulled in through the nose. Start by taking a deep inhalation, allowing the belly and ribs to softly expand, then sharply exhale, forcing all the air out by pulling the navel in toward the spine. As soon as all the air is pushed out, immediately relax your abdomen, pulling the air back in as you inhale. The technique is a bit tricky at first, and it might be helpful to place one hand over your navel to feel the contraction of your abdomen on your exhalations and its relaxation on your inhalations. Most important, try to stay relaxed overall. You should not experience tension in your shoulders, chest, or abdomen, just the rhythmic pulling and pumping of air. If you experience any unpleasant sensations such as dizziness or cramping, try slowing down and, if need be, take a few longer breaths. Women who are menstruating or pregnant should not do Breath of Fire.

In general, each exercise ends with a deep inhalation and a pause — holding your breath for a comfortable length of time while you apply the *bandhas* (body locks) — then a long exhalation as you completely relax in the pose. (Sometimes the teacher will instruct you to inhale, then to exhale and hold the breath out as you apply the body locks.) *Bandhas* are an integral part of the practice of Kundalini yoga. Also applied in meditation and at certain times during exercises, *bandhas* are energetic seals that contain and circulate *pranic* energy through the body and mind. However, although they work as dams in the subtle body, keeping the energy from flowing out of the body, the *bandhas* are applied physically by slightly contracting certain muscle groups and applying nerve pressure, increasing blood circulation in targeted areas of the body. When in place, the three main body locks — root lock (*mula bandha*), abdominal lock (*uddiyana bandha*), and throat lock (*jalandhara bandha*) — work together to lengthen the spine, keeping the *shushmana* open and the energy flowing up toward the higher *chakras* and brain centers. (For a full explanation of the application of the three main *bandhas*, please see chapter 4.)

Relaxation: The Art of Allowing

Miniperiods of relaxation are taken between exercises, so that the practice pulsates between active (doing) and passive (being). Upon your exhalation and release of the *bandhas*, rest comfortably in whatever position feels most natural at the end of each exercise (most likely sitting, kneeling, or lying either on your back or on your stomach with your head turned to one side). With your eyes still closed, relax as much as possible, keeping your awareness oriented inside. The easiest way to do that is to observe the natural rhythm of your breath. Be present to what you are experiencing within: Pay attention to what you are feeling and sensing, any thoughts or emotions that surface, without trying to do anything. Just be and allow whatever's taking place to run its course. The moment you start judging or try to manipulate what's happening, you miss the experience and the opportunity to tune in to the reality of what's actually occurring. Being that present in an expanded state of awareness, you are able to sense deeper levels of yourself and reality.

ALLOW YOURSELF TO LET GO

The invitation is to notice what feels comfortable and what feels out of place, being present to the sensations of your emotions, allowing yourself to experience whatever feelings arise. Stored negative thoughts and feelings will inevitably surface, and you may become frustrated or angry. While most of us try to avoid uncomfortable or painful emotions, they must be experienced — allowed and accepted with loving-kindness — in order to be released.

Relaxing between exercises, for ideally one minute, consolidates the effects of a *kriya*, allowing the biochemical, physiological, and energetic changes that occur to integrate within your body and psyche. It's crucial to allow the space and time for these changes to take place. You will most likely feel the general buzz of energy stirred up by the actions of the *kriya*. Over time, as you develop more mental focus, you will become more sensitive to the subtler sensations of energy, that is, its qualities, how it moves, where it's blocked, and so forth. The practice of Kundalini yoga not only stimulates *prana*, removing blocks in your subtle body and resistance in your psyche, but also raises the frequency of your energy, moving you into greater resonance with your true Self, or identity. The higher the vibration, the closer your innate energy is to aligning with universal energy, creating a conscious connection with the Divine.

The process of alignment is twofold: First, activation occurs, involving *kriyas* stimulating *kundalini*, opening the *chakras*, and pushing *pranic* energy through the *nadis*. Second, the process is simply allowed to unfold. Once free to move about, energy intuitively flows where it needs to go to promote healing and alignment, as long as there is no interference on your part. Therefore, these periods of "doing nothing" between yogic exercises are essential to the practice of Kundalini yoga. If you don't allow time for the energy to integrate and make the necessary adjustments, the exercises won't have nearly the same effect. After the allotted time, the teacher will instruct you through a deep inhalation and exhalation and into the next pose.

At the completion of a set, toward the end of class you will be guided into a longer period of relaxation (typically ten minutes or more), during which you will lie on your back in Corpse Pose. The approach is exactly the same — rest and do nothing but remain present and focused on the sensations you're feeling. Being able to simply relax is the first step in expanding your awareness, and you may find it difficult at first; even relaxing can take practice. Returning from relaxation, you'll be instructed to rotate your wrists and ankles, rub the soles of your feet and hands together, and place your palms over your eyes, breathing deep and relaxing the muscles of your face. After this you will lie on your back, curl into a ball, and rock up and down on your spine a few times, coming into a seated position to end practice in meditation.

Meditation is standard to all Kundalini yoga classes, as taught by Yogi Bhajan. The entire practice leading up to seated meditation prepares you for it. Not only do the *kriyas* bring the body and mind into a state in which meditation is easily fallen into, but you've also spent a considerable amount of class drawing your attention inward and developing your ability to remain present. All you need to do now is to still your body and focus on the meditation at hand. You can expect to learn a variety of techniques, the majority of which are accompanied by the internal chanting of *mantras*.

Hundreds, if not thousands, of meditations have been given by Yogi Bhajan, designed to change the biochemistry of the brain and transform the individual. There's a technique for just about everything, including meditations for healing, desire, trust, peace, a calm heart, to make the impossible possible, to heal the wounds of love, and so forth. Whatever the technique, Kundalini yoga practice followed by meditation brings the mind and body into an energetic state of balance — the springboard for spiritual development.

MEDITATE TO CLEANSE THE MIND

Whenever you sit quietly and turn your attention inward, you become aware of the sound track playing in the background of your mind. Oftentimes, especially in the early stages of your meditation practice, you will experience unpleasant or disturbing thoughts. And that's okay. Actually it's better than okay. As negative thoughts arise, the meditation technique is working to cleanse the mind.

Tuning In with *Mantras*

Chanting *mantras*, whether aloud or internally, is an integral part of Kundalini yoga practice, so much so that the style is often confused for "*mantra* yoga." *Mantras* are words, syllables, or phrases infused with psychospiritual powers that, when repeated, affect consciousness. Considered sacred utterances, they are energy-based sounds in ancient languages that have been passed down through certain yogic and spiritual lineages from master to initiated disciple. Believed to be expressions of elevated consciousness, *mantras* expand and deepen the mind, which then drops into the experience of infinite existence. The word *mantra* is loosely derived from the Sanskrit roots *manas* ("mind") or *man* ("to think") and *tra,* which denotes an instrument or tool, or *trana,* which means "liberation." *Mantras* are tools for calming and freeing the mind.

GURMUKHI *MANTRAS*

While *mantras* originated in the Vedas, ancient Indian Sanskrit texts, they are a customary practice within the traditions of Buddhism, Jainism, Sikhism, and Hinduism alike. Many of the *mantras* used in Kundalini yoga are taken from the Sri Guru Gran Sahib (Sikhism's religious text) and are chanted in Gurmukhi (the ancient Indian language of the Sikhs). But again, the practice of Kundalini yoga is not at all a Sikh religious practice.

The entire universe is made up of energy vibrating at various frequencies. Your thoughts, feelings, words, state of being — everything is a vibration of energy. Denser materials vibrate at lower frequencies, and higher frequencies resonate with spiritual connection and your true essence. Sound is a form of vibration; saying any word in any language generates a physical vibration. Sanskrit and Gurmukhi syllables carry powerful energetic vibrations; chant a particular sound and your body will resonate with that syllable's vibratory frequency. *Mantras* are actual tools for tuning in to, or accessing, specific vibratory frequencies. The many *mantras* within the Kundalini yoga tradition hold vibrations of peace, connection, prosperity, truth, and many other positive qualities, and when chanted they attract those very things to you (according to the law of attraction: frequencies attract one another). Ultimately, Kundalini yoga uses *mantra* to help create a vibrational connection with the Divine — merging the sound frequency of individual consciousness with universal consciousness, the highest vibration of all.

The science of *mantra* is quite fascinating. Chanting them clears the subconscious and directs the mind into higher vibrational frequencies by accessing different channels of your psyche through eighty-four pressure points, or meridians, on the roof of your mouth. Every time you speak or make a verbal sound, your tongue stimulates the nerves located in your upper palate, as well as the glands associated with them. *Mantras*, which are designed to tap out specific sequences, initiate a biochemical reaction that sends messages to the brain to open and activate the brain's higher centers. The science is basic reflexology of the tongue pressing the meridians on the upper palate. Different sequences clear the brain and deprogram the psyche. Tap the right "code" on the roof of your mouth and gain entry into your higher states of consciousness.

THE ESSENCE OF ALL SOUND

One of the primary goals of Kundalini yoga and *mantra* practices is tuning in to the eternal sound of the universe — the *naad*. Meaning "the essence of all sound," *naad* is the frequency fundamental to all languages throughout time. *Naad* is the cosmic sound that arises from one source or sound current. The universal sound current is the vibrational harmony of the infinite, uniting the individual self with the universal Self.

Every Kundalini yoga practice begins with chanting of the tuning-in Adi Mantra (*ong namo guru dev namo*, "I bow to the creative wisdom, I bow to the divine teacher within") three times. Unique to Yogi Bhajan's lineage, this *mantra* is designed to tune you in to the frequency of your highest spiritual consciousness, putting you in touch with your inner wisdom or teacher. Furthermore, chanting the Adi Mantra (*adi* meaning "primal" or "original") connects you to the link of Kundalini yoga masters, known as the Golden Chain, which protects and helps intuitively guide you as you practice the ancient technology.

Sat nam is the most basic and commonly used *mantra* in Kundalini yoga. *Sat* means "truth," and *nam* translates as "identity": *sat nam*, "truth is my identity." When you chant the potent affirmation, your entire being begins to resonate with the same vibratory frequency as your true identity and higher Self. The *mantra* is most often linked with the breath; you internally chant *sat* on your inhalation and *nam* on your exhalation. When another *mantra* is not specified, *sat nam* is chanted on the breath during almost all *kriyas*. (Don't worry if you don't catch on to this at first; chanting *sat nam* during class exercises will come naturally with continued Kundalini yoga practice.) Specific *mantras* given by Yogi Bhajan are also used in meditation to focus the mind and bring about certain beneficial physiological and psychological effects.

The Yoga of Awareness

Through the practice of Kundalini yoga and meditation, you begin to cultivate greater awareness of yourself on all levels of being. You progressively become more aware of your body, thoughts, and emotions, as well as your relationship with yourself, others, and the world at large. In a sense, you wake up. You notice more. You become more present to subtle differences and shifts, as well as to opportunities that may have previously escaped you. No longer living according to unconscious patterns or conditioned programming, you are able to consciously participate in creating the life you choose, empowered to make more daring decisions according to your inner destiny.

While you may not be in control of all life's circumstances, when you live consciously, you get to choose how you respond as situations present themselves. The more conscious you are of yourself, your internal motives, habitual patterns, emotional responses, and so forth, the more likely you'll respond and behave in ways that are the healthiest and best serve your higher Self. Once you're aware of what you are doing and why, you can choose to change your inner habits and outward tendencies. Conscious of your behavior and its impact, you act and speak with more mindfulness. Priorities become clearer as you begin to balance your inner and outer worlds. It's simple: Awareness affords you choices; choice is the gateway to freedom. Expand your awareness; experience more freedom.

INNER COMPASS

Kundalini yoga is about cultivating and following your inner guidance, the voice of your soul — your intuition. Yogi Bhajan taught that your intuition is your security. When you listen to your intuition, you know what to do. Following your intuition is the only way to ensure your happiness. Otherwise your life will be dictated by outside forces and influences.

As with all systems of yoga, the overriding goal of Kundalini yoga is union with the Divine. Also known as the "yoga of consciousness," Kundalini yoga is a powerful tool for facilitating greater levels of awareness. By expanding your awareness through the practice, you begin to cultivate a conscious experience of your highest Self, merging individual consciousness with universal consciousness, as well as getting in touch with your inner resources and gifts, so that you can discover the "sacred purpose in your life" and live accordingly.

Conclusion

There is nothing casual about Kundalini yoga; the practice, for those seriously interested in progressing or creating permanent change, requires discipline and commitment, as well as intention. A consistent daily *sadhana* (spiritual practice) is the foundation, heart, and soul of a Kundalini practitioner's life. Self-enriching, *sadhana* is a student's personal spiritual effort and is the method's main tool for working on the self and achieving one's higher purpose in life. *Sadhana* is a commitment to prayer, to clearing one's consciousness and relating to one's highest Self each morning before facing the world at large. Developing a deep *sadhana* practice, which should include exercise, meditation, and prayer, empowers you to live from a place of connection and authenticity as you take control of your life.

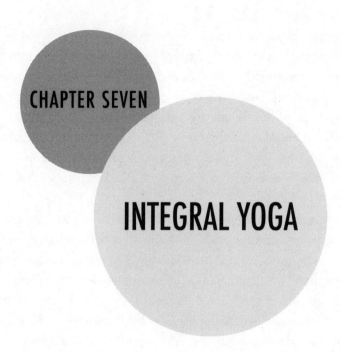

CHAPTER SEVEN

INTEGRAL YOGA

Integral Yoga is a flexible combination of specific methods designed to develop every aspect of the individual: physical, emotional, intellectual, and spiritual. It is a scientific system which integrates the various branches of yoga in order to bring about a complete and harmonious development of the individual.

— **SRI SWAMI SATCHIDANANDA**, founder of Integral yoga

Introduction: Truth Is One, Paths Are Many

Integral yoga is a comprehensive system that combines various yoga disciplines, *asana* practice, *pranayama*, meditation, *mantra* repetition, spiritual study, and selfless service, to develop every facet of an individual and his or her life. Classes are designed to address all layers of our being (known as *koshas* in Sanskrit), from the physical to the intellectual to the emotional, energetic, and spiritual, resulting in a relaxed body and calm mind. Students are gently guided to turn their attention inward and explore the effects of the postures and various yoga practices, bringing them more in touch with their body and mind, as well as their emotions and movement of subtle energy and, ultimately, with the deeper and more authentic aspects of their true Self. Transforming the whole person, Integral yoga aims to help students access the place of peace and happiness that resides within every individual and to live consciously from it.

The comprehensive lifestyle system was developed by one of the most renowned spiritual leaders of the twentieth century, Sri Swami Satchidananda (1914–2002). An Indian monk and dedicated disciple of Swami Sivananda, Satchidananda (affectionately known as Sri Gurudev) originally arrived in the United States for a two-day trip and ended up staying for a lifetime, spreading his essential teaching — happiness is our true nature and the birthright of every individual — throughout the West. With the slogan "Truth is one, paths are many," he touched the hearts of millions of people, believers and nonbelievers alike, from all walks of life throughout the world. Swami Satchidananda taught a combination of *hatha* yoga, meditation, chanting, and prayer as well as psychological, philosophical, and practical approaches to life, which he termed "Integral yoga." His approach was simple and direct, teaching ancient practices and spiritual lessons through storytelling and his own charming brand of witticism. He encouraged being of service to others, or *seva*, which became a fundamental tenet of Integral yoga. In addition to teaching *hatha* yoga classes, leading *kirtan* chants, and giving talks out of a large apartment on the Upper West Side of New York City in the late 1960s, he filled Carnegie Hall in 1969 with admirers, followers, and devotees who came to listen and learn from the great spiritual master. That same year Swami Satchidananda was invited to give the opening invocation at the original Woodstock Music and Art Festival, where he introduced chanting to hundreds of thousands of young people, telling them, "The entire world is going to watch this. The entire world is going to know what the American youth can do for humanity."

A SYNTHESIS OF YOGA TRADITIONS

The term *integral yoga* implies a synthesis of multiple yoga practices aimed at uniting, or integrating, all aspects of ourselves. There are two main schools of integral yoga, one developed by the renowned Hindu philosopher Sri Aurobindo, and the other founded on the teachings of Swami Satchidananda, which has been trademarked as Integral yoga in the United States. This chapter is concerned with Swami Satchidananda's Integral yoga, which is a combination of six branches of the yoga tradition: *raja* yoga, *hatha* yoga, *bhakti* yoga, *karma* yoga, *japa* yoga, and *jnana* yoga.

Soon Integral yoga teaching centers and institutes began popping up across the country, some of which included small residential communities where devotees could commit themselves to practicing and living the yogic path. Hundreds of Integral yoga teachers were trained, bringing the teachings of Swami Satchidananda to thousands of students in a variety of settings. His message resonated with those seeking greater meaning and depth than could be found in the superficial culture of American society at the time. They were after the lasting peace and happiness embodied in and promised by the influential swami. In August 1970 more than four hundred people attended the first Integral yoga interfaith retreat, held at Annhurst College, in Woodstock, Connecticut. Soon retreats were being held at multiple locations, attracting hundreds of people who were interested in experiencing *ashram* living. For up to ten days at a time, retreat attendees followed the same daily schedule as those followed by Integral yogis living in institutes and centers throughout the country (rising at dawn to meditate, engaging in the different yoga practices, and being of service).

As more and more students moved into the various Integral yoga institutes, Swami Satchidananda began sharing his vision for "Yogaville," a spiritual community where residents could grow their own food, educate their children, and devote themselves to the study and practice of yoga, as well as conduct commerce and create an economy established upon yogic values and guidelines. In 1972 Yogaville-West was established in Seigler Springs, California, followed by Yogaville-East one year later in Pomfret Center, Connecticut. However, by the end of the decade the Integral yoga community had outgrown both *ashram* sites, leading to the purchase of a much larger piece of property (totaling nearly seven hundred acres) in rural Virginia on the James River and the establishment of Satchidananda Ashram-Yogaville (SAYA) in 1979. Surrounding the *ashram* is the Yogaville community, consisting of private homes, a monastery for the monastic, dorms for guests and single residents, the Integral yoga school (Vidyalayam), various small businesses, an organic garden and orchard, and five sacred sites, including the LOTUS (the Light of Truth Universal Shrine). With over two hundred residents, SAYA is a unique, dynamic spiritual community of diverse individuals unified in their dedication to living the precepts of Integral yoga and a life of service. Each year thousands of guests visit Yogaville (the international headquarters of Integral yoga) to attend workshops, seminars, retreats, and teacher-training programs. For seekers and devotees, Yogaville is considered the happiest and most magical place on earth and continues to thrive on the teachings and essence of Swami Satchidananda, who entered Mahasamadhi (the state enlightened beings enter into upon making the final conscious decision to leave their physical body) while visiting India for a peace conference in August 2002.

THE LIGHT OF UNIVERSAL TRUTH SHRINE

The centerpiece of Yogaville, the LOTUS is a temple dedicated to interfaith understanding and harmony. Within the domelike structure, designed to replicate a lotus flower, are altars dedicated to the world's ten major religions as well as to faiths less well known and those unknown other than by the individual practicing them, totaling twelve. Opening in 1986, the shrine's two-day dedication ceremony held over the weekend of Guru Poornima was attended by religious leaders from all over the world. Sixteen years later, in 2002, the LOTUS was rededicated, becoming a memorial tribute to Swami Satchidananda.

Today there are six Integral yoga institutes in the United States, as well as one in Canada and one in India, and twenty-two centers world-wide, offering daily classes, intensives, and training programs. They also offer opportunities to learn more about a yogic lifestyle, including a vegetarian diet and ways to become involved in service activities; a few of the institutes offer small residential programs for those interested in deepening their commitment to a spiritual path. In general, classes, work-shops, and events are moderately priced or allow admittance by donation, ensuring that people from all income levels can receive the teachings and support they need to pursue their own lasting peace and happiness.

The Gist: Easeful, Peaceful, and Useful

Integral yoga involves a distinctly uncompetitive approach to *hatha* yoga that encourages students to work mindfully within their own comfort level and is therefore appropriate for all students regardless of age, ability, or degree of strength or flexibility. Teachers tend to be highly knowledge-able, especially those who have completed additional training programs, and can successfully adapt the poses and practices to all levels of ability. What's more, there are no expectations, and there's nothing to achieve as far as the physical experience or "look" of the poses is concerned. Instead of pushing and striving to prove anything to the teacher, or to themselves, for that matter, students are encouraged to practice the postures with an internal awareness — staying present to their physical ability and needs and working moderately from wherever that ability may be — and to let go of any preconceived notions of what they should be able to perform. More than a workout, Integral yoga is a "work in" designed to create an overall experience of healing, wellness, and peace that includes the body feeling relaxed and energized rather than spent from physical exertion. Classes tend to be gentle, slow, and accessible, placing equal emphasis on *pranayama*, deep relaxation, and meditation as well as *asana* practice. However, if you visit an Integral yoga institute or center, you will dis-cover a variety of classes from gentle yoga to exceedingly advanced lev-els, which introduce more difficult *asanas* and more advanced *pranayama* practices.

Upon taking your first class, expect to be welcomed. Integral yoga teachers are generally very warm and friendly, as well as very qualified to work with a wide population of students. The teacher will help you become situated and will most likely ask if you have any injuries or concerns before getting started. Class formally begins with a short opening chant followed by eye movement exercises, or yoga for the eyes. Many different chants (or prayers) are used in Integral yoga, chanting being a fundamental part of *japa* yoga (one of the six branches of yoga practiced in Integral yoga). The teacher will often give a brief explanation of the Sanskrit chant he or she has chosen for class so that students understand why they are chanting it and the meaning of its words, which are more about the feelings their sounds evoke than their actual definitions. The two most commonly used opening chants, however, are *om om om* (*om* being the primordial sound or vibrational hum of the universe) and *hari om* (the chant given by Swami Satchidananda at Woodstock). The chant goes as follows: *hari om, hari om, hari hari hari om,* and it is meant to energize your entire system. You'll also hear *hari om,* a common salutation in India, used as a greeting between Integral yogis. At the conclusion of the opening chant, there will be a few moments of silence before the yogic eye exercises are begun.

YOGA FOR THE EYES

While you are seated upright in a simple cross-legged position, the teacher will guide you through four eye movements: vertical, horizontal, diagonal, and full circles in both directions. After which, you will be told to rub your palms together and cup your closed eyes until they feel completely relaxed. Then you will be guided to lightly stroke your eyelids outward away from the bridge of your nose. Yogic eye exercises (*netra vyayamam*) increase circulation while relaxing the eye muscles, toning the optic nerve, and aiding in the general improvement of eyesight. They are especially beneficial for those who spend long hours on the computer or reading and writing.

Designed by Swami Satchidananda, Integral yoga classes are specifically set up to work from the grosser level, the physical body, down to the subtler layers of being, the emotional, energetic, and mental body. Every classical Integral yoga class follows the same format: warm-ups, *asana* practice followed by deep relaxation, *pranayama*, and meditation, concluding with a brief chanting session. *Asana* practice is used to strengthen and release tension in the physical body so the practitioner can become steady and relaxed. Working with the energetic level, *pranayama* not only energizes the whole system but also begins to draw the mind and senses inward in preparation for meditation. During meditation the body and mind become still, leading to an encounter with one's essence or true Self and highest potential. The overall aim of practice is to establish and maintain an "easeful body, peaceful mind, and useful life."

The physical part of class is generally forty-five to fifty-five minutes long, beginning with gentle movements such as cat-cow to awaken the spine, followed by a modified version of Sun Salutations, or Surya Namaskar, to further warm up all the major muscles and joints as well as increase circulation to all regions of the body. Next, the *asana* practice starts with standing poses common to almost all yoga styles, followed by a minimum of thirty seconds in Savasana, or Corpse Pose, as well as thirty seconds in a prone position (lying belly down) with arms resting alongside the body and palms up, before moving on to supine poses, seated postures, and twists. In beginning-level Integral yoga classes, more time is allocated for demonstrations and rest between the *asanas*; as you advance to level 2 and 3 classes, you will have fewer and fewer opportunities to rest, moving from one pose directly into the next as well as holding poses longer. Some Integral yoga flow classes are inspired by the *vinyasa* system; though they maintain the integrity and principles of classical Integral yoga classes, they are slightly more rigorous and faster paced. Regardless, the last half hour or so of any Integral yoga class will always be devoted to the subtler practices of *pranayama*, deep relaxation, and meditation.

Yoga Mudra, or Yogic Seal, is the last posture practiced in the *asana* routine. This involves sitting in a simple, comfortable cross-legged position with your spine erect and softly closing your eyes, taking a few easy, natural breaths, and directing your awareness within. Once you feel relaxed, you bring your hands behind your back and lightly grab hold of the right wrist with your left hand. Inhaling deeply, you slowly exhale as you hinge forward from the hips, keeping the spine as long as possible and coming as far forward as is comfortable. Eventually you will come to rest your forehead on the ground. Releasing all tension in the body, relax the breath and hold the pose for six or seven rounds of breathing, rising slowly on an inhalation. Then you sit quietly, resting your palms in your lap, and observe how you feel. Yoga Mudra (*mudra* meaning "gesture" or "seal") is meant to help the energetic transition from the physical practice to the subtler aspects of the full yogic routine, during which you are invited to reflect on your *asana* session and become deeply aware of your mental and physical state as a result of practice thus far.

Integral yoga classes include a period of deep relaxation (generally as long as fifteen to twenty minutes) known as yoga *nidra*, or "yogic sleep." This involves lying flat on your back with your legs loosely apart and arms at a comfortable distance from the body, palms facing up, and your eyes closed. The teacher will instruct you to raise, squeeze, and then abruptly release either the whole body at once or the major regions of the body individually. Once the entire body is relaxed and still, he or she will guide you to bring your awareness to each individual body part, beginning with the toes and soles of the feet, in order to mentally release any tension you may find. The process generally takes about five minutes, and once it's complete you'll be guided to observe the breath, without manipulating or controlling it in any way. Then you will be invited to observe your thoughts in the same passive manner, allowing anything that arises to be acknowledged, without identifying with each thought. Lastly, you'll be guided to notice that you are merely the observer of your breath and thoughts, resting easefully and effortlessly in your own peaceful self in a conscious state of deep sleep. After about five minutes of silence the teacher will guide the whole class back to a seated position for *pranayama* practice.

YOGA *NIDRA*

Yoga *nidra* is an essential practice in Integral yoga for calming the mind and integrating all the physical and physiological benefits of the preceding *asana* practice. Often referred to as a state of conscious deep sleep, yoga *nidra* helps release deeply held tension and unwind the autonomic nervous system, effectively reducing symptoms of stress and anxiety.

Common breathing exercises in Integral yoga include deep, or yogic, breathing, Kapalabhati (Skull Shining Breath), and Nadi Suddhi (Nerve Cleansing Breath). Helping to burn off any toxins released into the bloodstream during *asana* practice, *pranayama* is the essential precursor for meditation, bringing the breath, senses, and ultimately the mind under control. With the body and mind calm, steady, and relaxed, the last few minutes of class will be spent in meditation, usually accompanied by a *mantra*, followed by a closing chant of the teacher's choosing.

Meditative Approach:
Being Present, Attentive, and Accepting

Maintaining that true and lasting happiness can be attained only through right knowledge — that there is one infinite source of all life, that the essence of every living thing is but one spirit — Swami Satchidananda taught that one must transcend his or her limited personality to experience his or her true nature or Self (also known as God, the Divine, cosmic consciousness, Nirvana, and so on). In order to do so and to become a whole, mature person, one must fully develop and integrate every aspect of his or her self. Integral yoga is designed to facilitate an inward journey and the quest for self-knowledge. Each class is an opportunity to discover the depth of your own being, engaging all aspects of yourself, and, ultimately, come to know that place of profound peace, well-being, and stillness within.

There is an emphasis on finding a balance between effort and ease, challenge and comfort, during the *asana* portion of class (leaning more toward ease and comfort), so that the physical body still gets a nice workout without being overly aggressive or exerted. Beginning yoga students are advised to gently ease into their *hatha* yoga practice, releasing or coming out of the *asanas* before the natural breath becomes labored. Remember, there are no expectations as to what you can or should be able to do; the intention is to fully accept wherever you are in the pose without striving or straining to do more than what is comfortable. The primary focus of all Integral yoga classes is on being present, going inward, and opening up to the experience of the peace and joy that are always available within each of us. Instead of going into great detail about the physical alignment of the postures, teachers seek to create a supportive environment, providing clear-enough instructions and options for moving in and out of the *asanas* while promoting yoga's meditative qualities and cultivating a subtle inner awareness. More than anything, class is a time to be with yourself in a very attentive, accepting way.

THE GOAL OF INTEGRAL YOGA

"The goal of Integral yoga, and the birthright of every individual, is to realize the spiritual unity behind all the diversities in the entire creation and to live harmoniously as members of one universal family. This goal is achieved by maintaining our natural conditions of optimal health and strength, senses under control, a mind well-disciplined, clear, and calm, an intellect as sharp as a razor, a will as strong and pliable as steel, a heart full of unconditional love and compassion, an ego as pure as crystal, and a life filled with supreme peace and joy."

Within the Integral yoga system, alignment refers to the optimal flow of energy in the body. Unlike the aim of the systems of yoga that focus mainly on the anatomical alignment of the postures, the aim of Integral's more meditative approach to *hatha* yoga is to bring students in touch with their internal energy, or *prana*, ultimately allowing *prana* to direct the movements in and out of the *asanas*. Students are empowered to discover and learn for themselves, from within, where to place their muscles, bones, and joints, and as they advance from level 1 to level 2 and 3 classes, fewer and fewer instructions are given. Becoming quiet and listening to the teacher within are fundamental tenets of Integral yoga; following the inner movement of *pranic* energy, *asana* practice itself becomes increasingly meditative.

The tradition takes the same experiential approach to spirituality. Just as the teacher will not push you to work harder physically or command you to perform certain postures, he or she will not tell you what to believe and will not push anything spiritual down your throat. Integral yoga classes are very spiritual in nature; however, students are encouraged to adapt the teachings (or whatever is being taught, whether physical or philosophical), so that they are comfortable with the material presented, which can include completely ignoring any and all spiritual aspects of the practice. Teachers are there to serve you on your individual path of self-discovery in whatever form or fashion that suits you best. Grounded in the principles of peace, healthy and balanced living, and service, Integral yoga is open to all religions, faiths, and belief systems and respects the individual's right to choose his or her own path to lasting happiness. Rather than telling them what to believe, the system offers various ways and practices to help students have their own experience of their inner wisdom and peaceful truth.

A GENTLE INTRODUCTION

Integral yoga is rooted in classical yoga, *asana* and *pranayama* being only the third and fourth limbs of Patanjali's eight-limbed (ashtanga) yoga, and cannot be pulled out of and separated from the overall scope of yoga. Without sounding too preachy or forcing people to believe in certain concepts, Integral yoga teachers attempt to convey the much larger picture and more holistic objective rather than the physical benefits of *hatha* yoga alone and, in that way, begin to gently introduce yoga philosophy.

Six Branches of Yoga: Choose Your Own Way

While the aim of Integral yoga is the same as that of other styles — transformation of the whole person in pursuance of realizing the one spirit of all living beings — this style of yoga presents a variety of yoga practices for engaging, integrating, and developing all aspects of one's self. The idea is to find the combination of practices that appeal to you and suit your individual nature. The six main branches, or paths, of Integral yoga are *hatha* yoga (postures, breathing exercises, cleansing practices, and deep relaxation), *raja* yoga (concentration and meditation), *japa* yoga (repetition of *mantras*), *bhakti* yoga (love and devotion), *jnana* yoga (knowledge and wisdom), and *karma* yoga (selfless service), many of which are incorporated into the classical Integral yoga class described earlier. You may choose to dive deeply into one or all of the practices or simply attend weekly *hatha* yoga classes; the choice is yours, and all are welcome.

The eight-limbed path set forth by Sage Patanjali in his Yoga Sutras, *raja*, or royal, yoga is the foundation for all of the other branches of Integral yoga. Primarily concerned with stilling the mind in order for Self-realization to occur, *raja* yoga is a powerful tool for gaining self-mastery over all aspects of your life. However, most students don't start out in seated meditation, attempting to calm the activities of their mind; they begin first by working with the body to relieve stress and tension. In order for the mind to become calm and clear, the body must be healthy and balanced, *hatha* yoga being one of the most beneficial practices for the overall wellness of our physical, physiological, and subtle bodies. What's more, the mind-body connection established through *asana* practice helps to develop students' ability to concentrate and stay present from moment to moment, deepening their awareness and quieting their mind for meditation.

Hatha yoga is the physical approach to stilling the body and mind, whereas *jnana* yoga is the intellectual approach, or path of wisdom, to understanding our true nature through the attainment of knowledge. *Jnana* yoga students engage in scriptural study and self-examination, seeking answers to the most basic question of all: *Who am I?* Through a process of exploration, students begin to discover which of their attitudes, beliefs, and behavioral patterns, as well as relationships, are actually creating suffering and which are bringing joy. *Jnana* yoga appeals to those with an inquisitive nature, and engaging in it leads to the knowledge of Oneness and the direct realization of your true nature, which is limitless peace and joy.

Bhakti yoga, the path of devotion, is about cultivating a deep love and reverence for the Divine, or any name or form given to God. If you choose not to focus on an incarnation of the Divine, then you may focus on a spiritual teacher or truly any object of devotion that embodies your highest aspirations of lasting happiness. *Bhakti* yoga is the constant faith, remembrance, and worship of *something* that affirms your highest truth and oneness with everything in existence. By constantly serving something bigger than your small self, you begin to transcend your limited personality and view of the world to realize union with the universe. Providing an uplifting and healing path that is accessible to all, *bhakti* yoga practices include rituals centered on the object of devotion, chanting, prayer services, and other acts of worship big or small.

DEVOTIONAL WORSHIP

A *puja* is a ceremonial worship of a deity manifested in the form of an object, ranging from simple daily rites to elaborate temple rituals. This object of worship is meditated upon and then showered with offerings of flower garlands and petals, ghee, fruit, incense, and chants. In Integral yoga, a special *puja* is designed to invoke feelings of unity with all beings, using light, which is the universal symbol of all religions, as the main object of worship.

Considered a form of prayer, *japa* yoga is the concentrated repetition of a *mantra*, typically during meditation, though it can be performed during any activity. Again, the specific vibrations of the sound syllables of *mantras* represent various aspects of the Divine. By repeating a *mantra*, you begin to attune to the Divine vibration, connecting you to your highest Self. (For more information on the science of *mantra*, see chapter 6.)

One of Sri Swami Satchidananda's greatest teachings (and a core precept of Integral yoga) is that being of service, doing something for someone other than yourself, is the greatest joy in life. He said that, above all other branches or traditions of yoga, "*karma* yoga alone is enough to save your soul." *Karma* yoga is the path of selfless service. It is a path of action, of going, doing, and being out in the world, with absolutely no expectations or attachment to the results or outcome of your actions. Yoga teaches us that our expectations that situations will go a certain way or that we will receive something in return for our actions — if I do *a*, *b*, and *c*, then *x*, *y*, and *z* will happen — are what lead to anxiety, disappointment, and suffering. Life itself is full of successes and failures, agony and comfort, disasters and miracles. To remain completely detached from both desire and aversion is to be truly free — free to experience the peace that is always available at the core of your being. The fundamental concept is being selfless: taking any degree of selfishness or self-serving motivations utterly out of your actions.

Karma yogis live a life dedicated to serving the well-being of others. They are said to be "the conscious instrument of Divine Will." However, you don't have to quit your job or spend all your time and money doing charity work, though some *karma* yogis do. (For instance, Mother Teresa, the most renowned *karma* yogi, called her work "love in action.") *Karma* yoga is the path of living your everyday life in continuous dedication to the greatest good of all beings. More simply put, *karma* yoga is keeping an eye out for opportunities to help others, big or small: adding change to a stranger's expired meter, paying the toll for the car behind you, smiling at and making eye contact with a homeless person, paying someone a compliment in line at the grocery store, picking up random pieces of trash, calling a friend who just lost a loved one, dedicating your yoga practice to those who don't have the means to practice themselves, or saying a little prayer for those who are suffering. The opportunities are endless, but you have to look for them. Swami Satchidananda said that once you've tasted the real joy of helping someone else, "you won't want to miss the supreme joy of dedicated service."

Conclusion

In addition to offering daily *hatha* yoga classes, Integral yoga centers and institutes offer meditation and scripture study courses, weekly spiritual gatherings (*satsangs*), and *kirtan* (the art and practice of devotional chanting), as well as workshops on vegetarian diet and cooking, yoga philosophy and psychology, relationship and life skills, and a variety of other facets of a yogic lifestyle. For those interested in truly deepening their spiritual practice, Yogaville offers the Living Yoga Training (LYT) program, during which participants have the opportunity to fully immerse themselves in the teachings of Integral yoga and a yogic lifestyle for a minimum of one month, to participate in a variety of spiritual practices and service activities while living within a unique yoga community.

SATURDAY NIGHT *SATSANGS*

Derived from *sat*, meaning "truth," and *sanga*, meaning "community," *satsang* is a Sanskrit word meaning "gathering of seekers of the truth" or "in the company of the highest truth." A *satsang* is a gathering during which participants engage in a spiritual discussion led by a leader in the yoga community, often involving music, chanting, and prayer. *Satsangs* are traditionally held every Saturday night at Integral yoga institutes and at the Satchidananda *ashram*, Yogaville.

Many students find their way to Integral yoga institutes and centers in search of a more complete understanding of what yoga is and something deeper than the mostly physical experience offered in typical yoga classes. They like the holistic nature of Integral yoga. The system is also a great place to start if you are at all intimidated by the physical practice of yoga. The uncompetitive, no-expectations approach of Integral yoga classes is unmistakable, attracting gentler personality types of all ages and physiques. Bottom line, unless you're looking for a robust workout, you can't go wrong with Integral yoga, and you can expect to receive a well-rounded yoga education.

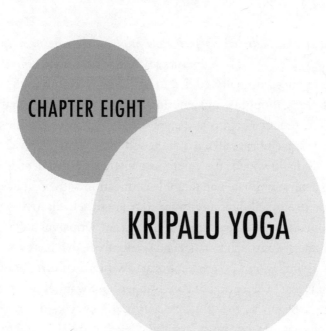

CHAPTER EIGHT

KRIPALU YOGA

Kripalu is the first traditional yoga *ashram* founded on the *guru*-disciple model to transition to a new paradigm of spiritual education. This paradigm is designed to provide tools that help individuals access their inner wisdom and find support for their ongoing process of growth and spiritual development. Kripalu honors all traditional and contemporary spiritual teachings that support the individual's direct experience of spirit.

— KRIPALU WEBSITE

Introduction: A Living Spiritual Tradition

Kripalu yoga is a comprehensive and compassionate approach to self-study that uses *asana*, *pranayama*, deep relaxation, and meditation as its primary tools for promoting physical health, calming the mind, opening the heart, and developing deeper levels of self-awareness. The method is inquiry based. Prompted by questions such as *What are you feeling right now? What is your body asking for? How might you create more space and softness in the pose? What is your heart saying? Where is your mind's attention?* students are continually guided to pay close attention to the internal urges, sensations, thoughts, and emotions flowing through them throughout class. The practice begins and ends with acceptance, a willingness to acknowledge and embrace all parts of the self in the light of consciousness. The aim of Kripalu yoga is for you to know yourself on a deeper level by cultivating a more intimate and tangible connection with what lies within. The method itself facilitates an inward journey of self-discovery.

Developed from the teachings of Swami Sri Kripalvananda, Kripalu yoga is a modern approach to yoga and spiritual life that has evolved over decades of assimilation into contemporary Western culture. Founded by Yogi Amrit Desai (a close and devoted student of Swami Kripalvananda), Kripalu yoga began as the Yoga Society of Pennsylvania, a nonprofit organization that offered yoga classes and teacher training and grew into an overflowing *ashram* community. In 1972, Yogi Desai, along with a few dedicated students, opened a residential yoga retreat in Sumneytown, Pennsylvania, with the intention of offering students a more complete yoga experience than the limited scope of a single class. During that time, Desai continued to travel back to India to study with Swami Kripalvananda and began adapting his guru's teachings into a secular format for his students in the States. Two years later the Yoga Society was renamed the Kripalu Yoga Fellowship to reflect the growing emphasis on the teachings of Swami Kripalvananda, and soon after, a second, much larger residential center was opened in Summit Station, Pennsylvania. Outgrowing both residential facilities, Kripalu purchased its current home at Shadowbrook (a former Jesuit seminary), in Stockbridge, Massachusetts, in 1983, which became the Kripalu Center for Yoga and Health. Led by Yogi Desai, who by then had assumed the mantle of spiritual leader and guru, the *ashram* living community flourished throughout the 1970s, '80s, and early '90s. At its height, as many as 350 full-time residents lived on-site. Some stayed for weeks or months at a time, and many others took up permanent residency in the *ashram*. Devoted disciples of Yogi Desai, community members went by Sanskrit names, donned all white, and upheld a strict *ashram* schedule, including yoga, *pranayama*, and meditation practice before dawn and countless hours of selfless service. They were a community of diverse individuals dedicated to living a spiritual life according to the fundamentals of the Kripalu tradition, which at that time included taking vows of celibacy.

SWAMI SRI KRIPALVANANDA

A renowned scholar, writer, and musician as well as a *kundalini* yoga master, Swami Kripalvananda devoted his life to awakening *prana* and spent a number of years living as a renunciant in India. In 1977, he moved to Pennsylvania to spend his last four years at the original Kripalu *ashram*, where he maintained his intense practice of *pranayama* and meditation for ten hours a day. The swami also gave occasional lectures there, serving as an example and providing teachings that inspired thousands of Western students to practice yoga regularly and live with compassion.

Under the guidance of Desai, the Western devotees began to assimilate the Eastern teaching they were studying and practicing. Leaders in the *ashram* community worked to develop a modest curriculum of yoga, holistic health, and self-discovery programs for the public to attend. By the 1980s Yogi Desai had become an international yoga figure and was traveling extensively, giving lectures, demonstrations, and seminars worldwide. Back at the Kripalu Center, senior residents were maturing into competent practitioners, leaders, and teachers in their own right. They started integrating yoga teachings and disciplines with growth psychology, current scientific and medical discoveries, and other modern approaches to personal development. Moving away from Sanskrit terms and ancient doctrines, they began transmitting the teachings of Kripalu yoga in clear language compatible with a Western worldview. An authentic spiritual tradition still rooted in the teachings of Swami Kripalvananda, Kripalu yoga was evolving into a new and contemporary format designed for students living active secular lives.

One of the major evolutions in the development of Kripalu yoga was the radical shift away from a guru-disciple paradigm to a new model of spiritual education that empowers students to learn from their direct experiences. In 1994, the tradition's guru-based decree unexpectedly imploded when Kripalu's spiritual leader, Yogi Desai, was ousted for engaging in inappropriate sexual relations with his students, among other exploits of dishonesty and abuse of power. The scandal shattered the Kripalu community, driving members to reevaluate the guru-disciple model the tradition was founded upon. Forced to resign, Yogi Desai left the *ashram*, and a group of senior faculty teachers and members were left to rebuild and restructure the Kripalu yoga system. What ensued was a new type of student-teacher relationship that avoids dependency and cultivates the capacity to learn from within. Now, rather than blindly following a guru, Kripalu students are taught through a process of self-inquiry to discover what is true for them according to their immediate experiences. Initially devastating, in the end Yogi Desai's sudden fall from grace proved to be a major catalyst for Kripalu yoga's unique model of experiential learning and nonsectarian approach to religious education. (Note: Yogi Desai, no longer associated with the Kripalu tradition, now teaches his own separate and distinct brand of yoga, Amrit yoga. Kripalu students are neither encouraged to study directly with Desai nor discouraged from it.)

EXPERIENTIAL EDUCATION

A completely undogmatic approach, Kripalu yoga encourages you to experiment on the mat and learn directly from your results, awakening you to your inner knowing and empowering you to make choices that are the best and healthiest for you in all facets of your life.

With the *ashram* dismantled, the remaining faculty and community leaders worked to reestablish Kripalu as a nationally recognized yoga retreat and experiential program center. Opening its doors to all spiritual disciplines and yoga traditions, the Kripalu Center now offers a wide array of classes, programs, types of training, workshops, and retreats with some of modern yoga's best-known instructors and leading holistic health and psychology professionals. The style's nonsectarian embrace of all styles and traditions of yoga, as well as its contemporary approaches to healing and self-discovery, is part of what makes Kripalu yoga unique and so effective as a method of personal and spiritual development. Considered a living spiritual tradition, Kripalu yoga continues to mature and deepen as it evolves and expands while remaining rooted in the foundation of Swami Kripalvananda's teachings of ethical living, regular yoga practice, compassionate self-acceptance, and attuning to the flow of *prana* in the body.

The Gist: Aspire to Be Present, Not Perfect

A highly creative system of yoga, Kripalu yoga can be adapted to fit the needs of all ages and ability levels. Neither *asana* sequences nor verbal instructions are standardized, giving teachers the freedom to apply the method to any form of yoga practice they desire. A Kripalu yoga class can look like a vigorous *vinyasa*-style flow, a slower-paced practice for seniors, or anything in between. Some Kripalu yoga teachers even teach hot, or Bikram-style, yoga classes, because they enjoy the athleticism and physical challenge. In fact, many teachers go through the Kripalu teacher training in order to learn the system's approach to self-discovery and the development of increased empowerment and personal choice, then go on to explore as well as teach other styles of yoga. What qualifies a class as Kipalu yoga is the methodology — the foundation from which the teacher teaches — rather than the form of practice.

At the heart of the Kripalu method lies compassion. (Swami Kripalvananda was named for the depth of his compassion, which he conveyed wholeheartedly through his teachings.) Kripalu yoga is a gentle approach to the practice of yoga that emphasizes compassionate self-awareness and acceptance. While recognizing the safety and importance of proper alignment, the approach doesn't strive to perfect the structure of the postures; there's really no right or wrong way of doing the poses in Kripalu yoga. The method is more malleable than other styles of yoga in terms of the teacher's approach to individuals, which invites students to check in with "where they are" each time they step onto the mat and to honor their body's needs and limits. Guided to ask questions, such as *What happens if I widen my right foot* or *shift my weight to the left?* students are encouraged to move and modify the postures until the position feels just right for them. Teachers are there to lead you through the postures, offering skillful instruction and compassion while also encouraging self-sourcing. There's an unmistakable exploratory nature to Kripalu yoga that you won't find in most other yoga classes, requiring students to have a bit more patience and the desire not only to know themselves but also to know what's best for them in every moment of their lives.

PRACTICE WITH COMPASSION

Kripalu yoga's compassionate approach is often misinterpreted as "gentle yoga," which is simply not the case. The style encourages students to respect their body's limitations while learning not only how to work within it but how to expand it as well. Experienced teachers will be able to hold a compassionate space, allowing each student to explore the poses in his or her own way while encouraging and inspiring students to push themselves and work through challenging moments. That being said, if you're interested in being drilled through a vigorous workout, Kripalu yoga isn't the style for you.

Integrating traditional Eastern beliefs and disciplines with contemporary therapy approaches and understandings, Kripalu yoga uses yoga techniques that activate *pranic* energy in the body together with awareness-focusing techniques that foster healing and growth, as outlined in three stages: *body and breath awareness, holding the postures,* and *meditation-in-motion.* Beginning with the *practice of being present,* each stage is designed to access progressively higher levels of self-awareness, bringing you into contact with your own consciousness. As your sensitivity and receptivity heighten and you're able to feel and notice more, you become increasingly aware of the thoughts, emotions, sensations, and feelings continuously flowing through you as you practice. In class, students are repeatedly invited to pause, breathe, relax, feel, and watch everything that arises, with an attitude of acceptance. The practice is to simply observe and allow whatever's happening in the moment, cultivating the ability to remain present to your inner experiences with unjudgmental awareness.

Stage 1 methodology teaches students how to be fully present in their body by willfully applying alignment and breathing techniques. Emphasizing the physical practice of yoga postures, the first stage of Kripalu yoga strengthens and purifies the body, building a strong container for increasing *pranic* energy in the later stages. Stage 2 methodology develops students' ability to "stay with it" and sit with whatever feelings, thoughts, and emotions surface. Postures are held for extended lengths of time as students deepen their mind-body connection and attune to the inner flow of sensation and energy. Opening the heart and clearing the mind, the second stage of practice awakens *prana* in the body, which can be felt as an electric-like current, a tingling, or a warm sensation. Once awakened, the intelligent energy of *prana* guides every movement of the body in the next and final stage of Kripalu yoga, and practice becomes a very personal moving meditation.

PRANA: SOURCE ENERGY

A key understanding of the practice of Kripalu yoga is that all thoughts, emotions, sensations, and impulses are sourced by *prana*. If the body's *prana* is blocked or unstable, thoughts and emotions are chaotic and unbalanced. Attuning to the flow of source energy naturally brings all levels of your being into harmony.

Kripalu yoga classes generally begin with students bringing themselves present, settling into their space, and connecting to their breath. Individual teachers may lengthen this centering process, choosing to read a poem or a passage to impart a simple spiritual teaching. A *pranayama*, or breathing exercise, is almost always incorporated into the beginning of class, followed by gentle warm-ups before the *asana* portion of practice. The *asana* portion promotes a balanced sequence of postures with a considerable focus on strengthening the core muscles of the torso (belly, chest, and back), which are weak in most people and are needed to support the proper alignment of the spine. Referred to as a "yoga flow" in Kripalu yoga, a skillfully planned sequence unfolds the poses in a way that intuitively makes sense to the body, moving from basic to more challenging postures and cooling down with movements that are calming and integrative. Meant to be extremely rejuvenating, each class concludes with deep relaxation (or yoga *nidra*).

Relaxation is an essential component of the Kripalu yoga method. The combination of postures and deep breathing in conjunction with relaxation, which comes naturally after *asana* practice, releases tension, calms the mind, and restores the nervous and endocrine systems, ultimately bringing the body back to a healthy state of balance. Kripalu teachers will almost always leave at least ten minutes at the conclusion of class to lead students into a deep relaxation using a combination of different techniques. Lying in Corpse Pose, or Savasana, you will be guided to release the full weight of your body onto the floor beneath you. Begin by allowing the breath to return to its natural state. As you let the breath flow freely in and out, gradually lengthen your exhalations until they are about twice as long as your inhalations. This kicks in the parasympathetic nervous system, inducing the relaxation response. Next, the teacher will most likely guide you through progressive relaxation, so that you systematically release tension muscle by muscle until your entire body is completely relaxed. When through, the teacher will gently guide you back from the profound state of rest, inviting you to take as much time as you need. Instead of saying *namaste*, which is the common expression used to close most yoga classes, essentially meaning "the light in me bows to the light in you," the teacher will use *jai bhagwan*, an interchangeable Hindi term.

Stage 1: Willful Practice

Stage 1 methodology uses mental focus, alignment details, and breath-movement coordination to develop and increase awareness of the body and breath. Often called "willful" practice for its emphasis on external techniques, Kripalu yoga's first stage teaches students how to intentionally structure the classical yoga postures according to simple alignment principles. The ongoing language around body awareness directs students' attention to what they're physically attending to in the poses, requiring them to be fully present. Movements naturally slow down as you consciously flow through the postures, pausing from time to time to attune to the sensations taking place in your body before moving on to the next pose.

THE PRACTICE OF BEING PRESENT

The *practice of being present* is Kripalu yoga's core technique, which you will start to become familiar with in your very first class.

BREATHE: Consciously deepen your inhalations and exhalations.

RELAX: Soften and let go of any muscular tension.

FEEL: Open to the experience of sensations.

WATCH: Closely observe what's taking place without grasping or denying.

ALLOW: Accept every part of yourself and your experience as it is.

Sustaining an even-flowing breath is essential to the practice of being present. In yoga we learn that the breath and mind and emotions are intricately related: When the mind is agitated by fear, stress, or anger, breathing becomes shallow and erratic; when the mind is focused and calm, breathing flows freely and evenly. Consciously breathing slowly and smoothly soothes and clears the mind, restoring emotional balance. An even-flowing breath helps you stay present on your mat. Referred to as "ocean-sounding breath," the breath moves rhythmically in and out through the nostrils, while inhalations and exhalations are synchronized with the motions in and out of the poses. Slower movements help you establish an even-flowing breath, which will continue to lengthen and deepen with practice.

Kripalu yoga simplifies postural alignment with *press points*. Using basic language and as few words as possible, teachers instruct students to press into specific body parts (or points) as they build, hold, and release the pose with awareness. Commonly used press points include the four corners of the feet, the sitz bones, the crown of the head, the pubic bone, the tailbone, the sides of the hips, the tops of the shoulders, and the shoulder blades. Engaging specific press points in a pose quickly brings the body into alignment, freeing the mind from having to hold a conglomeration of anatomical details so that students can focus on what they are feeling in their body. Encouraged to investigate their body's response to the various press points and experiment with making subtle adjustments while practicing with alignment, students can safely explore the poses within the healthy limits of their body's flexibility and range of motion. Kripalu yoga's simple approach to body alignment allows students to shift out of their intellectual thinking center and into their feeling center. As presence deepens on the mat, your sensitivity heightens, and you become increasingly aware of the way your body *feels* in a pose, as well as becoming aware of any internal urges, which you are encouraged to follow.

BASIC PRINCIPLES OF ALIGNMENT

When you stay present and work with press points, the basic principles of alignment become part of your body's felt-sense.

- Build the posture from the ground up.
- Stabilize the core.
- Elongate the spine.
- Open the chest, position the shoulders.
- Keep the neck an extension of the spine.
- Position the limbs.
- Hold and release with awareness.

Stage 2: Will and Surrender

Stage 2 methodology is designed to steadily heighten students' moment-to-moment awareness of the sensations, emotions, and thoughts as they emerge throughout practice. Practicing with eyes soft or shut, students hold poses for longer periods of time to facilitate an inward focus as they learn to shift their attention from the alignment of the postures to what's taking place on the inside. Guided to remain focused on the felt-sense of their body, students are encouraged to listen to the body's internal prompting and follow any impulses to move or make sounds (audible exhalations, sighs, even moans) as they arise. Micromovements (small, natural, slow-motion movements) are used in the postures to investigate minor variations and discover new ways in which the body wants to move and open, releasing tension in the broader regions. The invitation to pause between long holdings allows students to relax and let go on a deeper, subtler level before moving on to the next pose. Stage 2 practice cultivates an intimate, nurturing relationship with your body. Learning to adhere to internal promptings and urges, you begin to develop an intuitive sense of what your body needs.

Rather than powering or struggling through a challenging posture, students can use a technique for holding poses that allows them to relax and breathe deeply while they explore micromovements. One of the core components of stage 2 practice is *finding the edge* — that optimal place where the stretch is neither too much nor too little. Practicing at your edge allows you to make steady gains in flexibility without placing unnecessary strain on the muscle fibers and joints. Practicing short of the edge, you're doing yourself a disservice; beyond the edge, you're running the risk of injury. On the brink of discomfort, your mind naturally focuses, allowing you to enter the subtlety of your inner experiences.

METAPHOR FOR LIFE

Holding a pose for a prolonged length of time is just as much a test of inner strength as it is of physical strength. Practicing at the edge you will encounter your self-perceived limitations. The invitation is to work with them, respecting your body's limits while also transcending them. Simply holding a pose one or two breaths longer than what you think you're capable of handling allows you to access your inner strength and move beyond the preconceived limitations that your mind places on you.

If you hold a pose long enough, who knows what will come up on the different layers, or *koshas*, of the body. Inevitably, buried, often painful emotions and psychological tension will surface during stage 2 practice. That's what holding the postures with heightened awareness is designed to do: unearth unconscious material, allowing deep-seated emotions, stress, and perceptions (self-limiting thoughts and beliefs) to materialize on the mat, where they can be experienced and let go. Creating a supportive environment and encouraging self-compassion, Kripalu yoga teachers facilitate an inward journey that allows students to explore all aspects of themselves without judgment. The method teaches students how to compassionately embrace the full spectrum of their experiences, encouraging them to accept and attend to whatever arises during practice by allowing themselves to fully feel the sensations of their emotions as well as acknowledge their thoughts with loving compassion.

Two new techniques are introduced in the second stage of Kripalu yoga to support the inner work taking place: *riding the wave* and *witness consciousness*. The first technique, riding the wave of your moment-to-moment experience, is Kripalu yoga's unique approach to emotional release. As you hold the posture, begin by noticing any sensations you may be experiencing in your body. Your attention will naturally be drawn to the area where sensation is felt the strongest; focus there, immersing all of your awareness in the feeling. Energy builds in the body with concentration, increasing the benefits of the pose. As layers of stress are released and stored emotions and mental tension emerge, a powerful wave of sensation will begin to swell in your inner body. Resist the tendency to deny, "fix," or even understand the feelings and thoughts you encounter. Remain focused on the strong sensation and continue to consciously relax and breathe, allowing the wave to build in intensity. Surrender to the experience and stay absorbed in the felt-sense of emotions and the energy in your body. Watch as the feelings and energy of sensations shift and change. Eventually the wave will crest and dissipate. For the student who commits to staying present and truly feeling whatever surfaces, even if the experience is uncomfortable, trapped emotions, stored traumas, and mental disturbances will be released. But you have to go through it: You must experience your feelings and acknowledge your thoughts without judgment in order for them to be released and for emotional healing and psychological growth to take place.

EMOTIONS WELCOMED

While many spiritual traditions discourage strong emotions, considering them to be distractions or impediments to practice, Kripalu yoga welcomes and honors all emotional experiences as potent catalysts for growth. The tradition recognizes the transformative energy behind all emotions and encourages students to never avoid or reject painful emotions, which bring important messages to the forefront of your consciousness.

Although it can be very disconcerting at first, staying rooted in the moment-to-moment experience of strong sensations and emotions, without denying or attempting to manipulate them, leads to what the Kripalu tradition calls "witness consciousness." The practice of being fully present in your body gradually matures into a state of unjudgmental awareness that allows you to objectively observe without reacting to or attaching value to what comes up. Witness consciousness enables you to remain fully present in a state of meditative awareness without being distracted by the steady stream of thoughts, emotions, and sensations flowing through you. Stage 2 practice teaches students how to stay immersed in the reality of their inner experiences without input from the judging mind and also without avoiding uncomfortable thoughts and emotions or grasping at what's enjoyable. No longer denying your emotions, thoughts, and perceptions or deeming them as bad or good, pleasurable or painful, worthy or unworthy, you can begin to recover, acknowledge, and embrace all parts of yourself in the light of consciousness. A new clarity emerges beyond the conditions of the mind. Witness consciousness affords you, as the observer, the necessary distance to begin to recognize the deeper truths not only of your experiences but also of your existence, leading to the discovery of who you truly are.

Stage-two practice lies right on the cusp of will and surrender. While still consciously building and holding the postures, students begin to deepen their internal awareness, surrendering to whatever arises. When students remain present with compassionate awareness — acknowledging, accepting, and allowing tension, fears, and unconscious restrictions to surface — emotional and mental blocks begin to dissolve, releasing *prana* to move freely through the body. Attunement to the inner flow of *prana*, which animates and regulates every function of the body and mind, initiates a natural and steady process of healing at all layers of your being.

Stage 3: Surrender to the Wisdom of the Body

Everything learned and practiced willfully in the previous stages — all alignment and breathing techniques, rules, and restrictions — is dropped in the third and final phase of Kripalu yoga. The entire practice is guided from within: Every movement on the mat is in direct response to the body's instinctive impulses without interference from the mind. Stage 3 methodology is designed to cultivate a deeper awareness of the body's *prana*. Sustaining an inward focus, absorbed in the feeling of sensations, you begin to allow the inner flow of energy to move your body. Postures spontaneously emerge according to your body's intuitive wisdom. One pose naturally dissolves into the next as awakened and uninhibited *prana* guides the movements with an innate intelligence that knows exactly what the body needs in every moment.

Yoga postures take on a new depth when you surrender to the wisdom of the body. Seamlessly flowing in and out of postures in a state of inner absorption, your yoga practice becomes a form of *meditation-in-motion* (Kripalu yoga's hallmark). A highly personal experience, practice deepens as you attentively attune to the inner flow of source energy. Sensations become more distinct, mental awareness grows more refined, and *prana* builds in the body, leading to what Kripalu calls "yoga experiences." Compelling and revelatory, yoga experiences (or peak experiences, as they are referred to in psychology) offer you momentary glimpses into your true nature, leading to the profound realizations and awakenings yoga is intended to generate. As you cultivate an intimate relationship with your inner world, you'll inevitably encounter yourself in new ways and capacities beyond the ordinary manners in which you're used to experiencing yourself. Whether you feel your body release on a deeper level, are called to rely upon your inner strength, have a powerful insight, or become deeply absorbed in the breath and sensations, your perception of yourself shifts (if only for a moment). Yoga experiences expand your awareness of who you are and what you are capable of handling and achieving. Transitional phenomena, these moments of expanded awareness serve as potent catalysts for growth and change, freeing up more creative energy in the body — ultimately transforming your sense of self.

The experience of meditation-in-motion can be entered into from stage 1 or 2, using any of the techniques outlined in the previous sections, or from what the Kripalu tradition refers to as "posture flow." Sitting quietly relaxed with a conscious flowing breath and inward focus, you begin posture flow when you feel the urge to move. If one arises, follow it. Allow *prana* to gently guide your body into movements and positions without interfering with the impulses to move in a certain way or making an effort. If the impulse to move never emerges, begin by initiating a slow, simple movement and let it continue to flow until you feel it come to a natural stop. As practice deepens, you will become increasingly sensitive to the promptings of *prana* to move the body, and posture flow will become a natural outpouring of your yoga practice. Often described as a moving prayer invoked by a deepening connection to *prana*, the third phase of Kripalu yoga brings you into direct contact with spirit as the intelligent, animating force of the body, mind, and emotions.

THE THREE STAGES OF KRIPALU YOGA

A mature-depth practitioner will seamlessly pass through all three stages of Kripalu yoga in one session on the mat. Willfully warming up and becoming present in the body, the practitioner holds poses to facilitate an inward awareness and release tensions as he begins to attune to the sensations of *pranic* energy and to allow micromovements and sounds to spontaneously emerge. The flow of *prana* then guides him into intermittent periods of moving meditation. Once free-flowing movements come to a natural stopping point, the process begins again as he willfully forms a new pose before surrendering once again to the innate wisdom of *prana* to direct the body.

Path of Transformation

The three stages of Kripalu yoga set forth a path of transformation that facilitates physical and emotional healing, psychological growth, and spiritual attunement. As layers of stress, pain, resistance, and tension dissolve, physical vitality, mental clarity, and emotional stability emerge, leading to a series of insights and positive changes that awaken you to realize your full potential. You begin to look at yourself and your life with new transparency and an increased capacity to accept things as they are with more empathy and compassion for yourself and others. Regular practice helps you access your inner knowing and strength, allowing you to live with a stronger connection between your outer self and what lies within you. No longer living according to social conditions or external guidance, you begin to respond to life's circumstances with more authenticity and awareness, which increases your personal choice and empowers you to make decisions that support your deepest identity and aspirations.

THE GIFT OF PRESENCE

By learning to allow whatever's happening on the mat and just be with it, you develop the capacity to be fully present in every moment of your life. The true gift of Kripalu yoga is living wholly present, experiencing life to its fullest — allowing life itself to touch and transform you.

Central to the understanding of the tradition's approach to personal and spiritual development is the radical stance that *all is well* — that you are already worthy, complete, whole, and intrinsically connected to spirit. Using the tools of yoga to free the inner flow of *prana* in the body, Kripalu yoga was designed to remove the blocks that keep you from experiencing the reality of who and what you truly are. Attuning to source energy, you touch the core of your being, causing a sudden and profound shift in your consciousness. You awaken to your true Self. Swami Kripalvananda described the process of spiritual attunement as a "journey from the known to the unknown." The three stages of Kripalu yoga facilitate that journey, taking you into the depths of your being and into direct contact with your own source energy, forging a living relationship with spirit.

Conclusion

In the end, Kripalu yoga is a spiritual practice that extends well beyond the mat to create a holistic lifestyle founded on the principles of yoga. And while taking your yoga "off the mat" isn't a concept exclusive to Kripalu yoga, Kripalu is one of a few systems to make "living your yoga" its primary focus. The system attracts and supports those who desire to transform all or some part of their life. It's about being awake and present in every moment of your life, listening to the wisdom of your body, and making healthy, conscious choices for yourself.

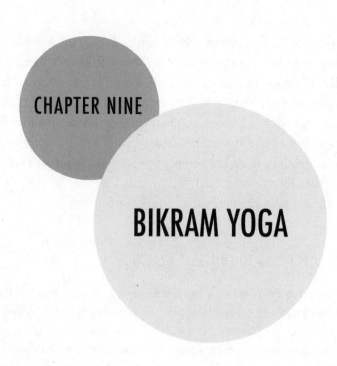

CHAPTER NINE

BIKRAM YOGA

Your mind is your number one enemy. When you come to my class I guarantee you, for 90 minutes you will forget who you are, what is your name, whether you are man or woman, what you are doing here; for the first time since you were born your mind will be totally free, meditated from the rest of the world: I take you to another galaxy.

— **BIKRAM CHOUDHURY,** founder of Bikram yoga

Introduction: Welcome to Bikram's Torture Chamber

Consisting of twenty-six postures and two breathing exercises done in 105-degree heat with 40 percent humidity for ninety minutes, Bikram yoga is going to challenge you on every level of your being. Quite unlike any other physical experience, the practice demands everything you've got: all of your muscles, strength, concentration, and willpower. Physical, mental, and emotional stress pours out with every rivulet of sweat, leaving you completely relaxed and "energized from the inside out." The sequence of twenty-six yoga *asanas*, selected by Bikram Choudhury, systematically works every part of the body from "bones to skin," bringing fresh, oxygenated blood to every internal organ, vein, gland, fiber, and other tissue in order to restore and maintain optimum health and maximum function of all bodily systems. In ninety minutes, Choudhury promises, his scientifically designed series of twenty-six poses will strengthen, relax, reshape, restore, and heal "all of you," as long as you follow his instructions and give 100 percent of your effort.

TWENTY-SIX POSES TO COMPLETE HEALTH

Stripping away the overtly spiritual and dogmatic components of the yoga tradition, Choudhury isolated twenty-six "medicinal" yoga postures and two breathing exercises for their therapeutic value — specifically their value to the sedentary Western lifestyle, which has created sluggish organs and poor posture from excessive sitting and computer use. In his manual, *Bikram's Beginning Yoga Class*, Choudhury declares that medication, surgery, or even regular exercise fails to heal what ails America. "What you are looking for is my beginner's yoga class."

Over years of application and research Choudhury developed a series of *asanas* that has the potential to cleanse, heal, and strengthen the body no matter how old, sick, tired, or injured a person may be. A one-size-fits-all method, Bikram yoga has attracted thousands of followers who resoundingly confirm its ability to restore physical vitality and enhance overall well-being, as well as cure a variety of chronic health conditions. Testimonies of the style's therapeutic benefits circulate throughout studios and the larger Bikram yoga community, including the series' ability to heal knee and spinal disk injuries, reverse diabetes, lower blood pressure, improve digestion, stop migraines, cure autoimmune diseases, lift depression, and reverse arthritis and osteoporosis. Choudhury has created an empire selling the healing attributes of *hatha* yoga, claiming that you will live a stronger, healthier, longer, and more peaceful life just by practicing his method the right way.

Choudhury also makes the bold claim that Bikram yoga is the only authentic form of classical *hatha* yoga being practiced in the West. Having learned the eighty-four original classical yoga postures from his guru Bishnu Ghosh (one of India's most celebrated physical culturists and, according to Choudhury, the highest authority on classical *hatha* yoga), Choudhury devised a style that remains true to the way the postures were performed thousands of years ago. Following three basic principles — freezing (or holding) the body in a posture for a prescribed length of time, properly controlling the breath while in the pose, and following each *asana* with the minimum twenty seconds of complete relaxation in Savasana — Choudhury asserts that his method is the only correct way to practice *hatha* yoga. And unless you practice the right way (exactly as he teaches the *asanas*), you will not receive the benefits of doing the yoga posture.

Born in Calcutta, India, in 1946, Choudhury began practicing yoga at the age of four. He attended Ghosh's College of Physical Education in Calcutta, where he practiced yoga for four to six hours every day, and won the National India Yoga Competition in three consecutive years, retiring at the age of sixteen as the undisputed All-Indian National Champion. Also an accomplished runner and weightlifter, Choudhury injured his knee one year later in a weightlifting accident, which doctors predicted would leave him crippled for life. Refusing to accept that he would never walk again, Choudhury returned to Ghosh's college and, under the guidance of his guru, completely recovered from the knee injury in six months. Ghosh then sent him to Mumbai to teach and help sick people in one of the world's most populated cities. At the time yoga was traditionally taught one-on-one, teacher to disciple; however, upon arriving in Mumbai, Choudhury discovered that there were more sick and debilitated people than he could help on an individual basis. Boiling the eighty-four postures learned from his guru down to twenty-six, he designed a sequence of *asanas* that would help large groups of people regardless of their condition or ailment. Thus the Bikram yoga series was born.

YOGENDRA BISHNU CHARAN GHOSH

Bishnu Ghosh was the younger brother and first disciple of Swami Yogananda, author of the acclaimed *Autobiography of a Yogi* and founder of
the Self-Realization Fellowship. Passionate about scientifically documenting
the healing attributes of *hatha* yoga, Ghosh opened his College of Physical
Education in 1923 and developed health and fitness methods based on the
eighty-four classical *asanas*.

At the urging of Ghosh, the Indian yoga master arrived in Beverly
Hills, California, in the early 1970s and founded Bikram's Yoga College
of India. Teaching mostly athletes and Hollywood stars, such as Kareem
Abdul-Jabbar and Elizabeth Taylor, Choudhury quickly gained a widespread reputation for healing through his series of twenty-six postures,
and he began attracting a loyal foundation of students and devotees. However, it wasn't until he started offering his intensive teacher training, at the
urging of his wife, Rajashree Choudhury (herself a five-time All-Indian
Yoga champion), in 1994 that Bikram yoga's popularity exploded across
the country and throughout the world. An equally prominent figure in the
Bikram yoga community, Rajashree helped design the certification process and proved to be a strong businesswoman, bringing a soft presence to
the Bikram organization in contrast to Choudhury's harsh teaching style.
Eight years later, he copyrighted his series of twenty-six yoga poses and
two breathing exercises, much to the dismay and outrage of the larger yoga
community, and began franchising his style of yoga. Everything under
the Bikram yoga name has since been trademarked, including Bikram hot
yoga and Bikram's Yoga College of India.

CELEBRITY STATUS

Self-proclaimed guru to the rich and famous, Choudhury poses in photos
with his celebrity students, including Ted Kennedy, President Clinton, Indira

Gandhi, and Shirley MacLaine, which cover the high walls of the Bikram Yoga International Headquarters, in west Los Angeles. Still more celebrities, including Madonna, Lady Gaga, Jennifer Aniston, and David Beckham, frequent the Bikram yoga headquarters.

Choudhury states that the copyrights and trademarks serve to preserve the Bikram yoga method, which must be taught in a very specific way that requires appropriate training and knowledge to effectively teach. He sees his legal dominion over this style of yoga, which has grown from about ten studios in 1996 to more than six hundred worldwide today, as an issue of quality control, and he personally certifies all of his instructors, who must complete an intensive nine-week training course requiring five hundred hours of study and (in 2013) costing between $11,400 and $15,500 with mandatory hotel accommodations. Led by Choudhury, Rajashree, and their staff of senior teachers, the course covers anatomy, *asana*, nutrition, the therapeutic applications and health benefits of yoga, the philosophy of yoga, and the Bikram yoga dialogue (yes, there is a script). Teachers are expected to memorize the dialogue, reciting it verbatim in every class, ensuring that everyone who takes Bikram yoga is following the exact instructions of Choudhury himself (and thus doing the *asanas* "the right way"). Teachers who complete the training have a thorough understanding of the Bikram method and receive support in setting up and marketing their own Bikram yoga studio (for an initial franchising fee of $10,000 as well as a monthly royalty). Since the style has exploded in popularity, "hot yoga" classes have begun popping up everywhere. Although similar, hot yoga is not Bikram yoga. Just to be clear: Bikram yoga can be practiced only under the guidance of a Bikram-certified instructor at a Bikram-affiliated studio (otherwise known as "Bikram's torture chambers"), which are specifically designed and built to facilitate the proper heating and climate necessary to practice the Bikram yoga series.

YOGA'S BAD BOY

Bikram Choudhury has attracted a wealth of media attention (and naysayers) for copyrighting centuries-old *asanas* and his claim to cure all in twenty-six poses. Since arriving on the American yoga scene in 1973, he has earned the reputation as the "bad boy of yoga" for his egocentric behavior (most notably his heavy collection of Rolexes and Rolls Royces), excessive franchising fees, and numerous lawsuits he's filed against those who infringe upon his intellectual property rights, not to mention the various sexual harassment suits filed against him.

The Gist: Bikram's Beginning Yoga Class

Bikram yoga is instructional-based *hatha* yoga designed for beginning students, so that students at any level of experience can attend the same class and practice the same series of poses regardless of age, ability, ailment, or level of fitness. The scripted dialogue that accompanies every class is specifically geared toward someone who has never practiced yoga *asana* before, giving verbal instructions on how to enter, hold, and exit the postures. Each pose is explained in detail, including the posture's medical benefits as well as problems you may encounter, clues for making rapid progress, and even ways in which you might be enticed to cheat in an *asana* and therefore deprive yourself of the posture's full benefits. The dialogue is meant to keep you engaged in the moment, requiring that you remain focused and listen to the teacher's precise instructions in order to perform the pose correctly.

Performing the pose "correctly" in Bikram yoga does not mean perfect execution. Receiving the benefits of the *asanas* does not require that they be performed perfectly. Instead, Bikram yoga emphasizes "trying the right way." Choudhury stresses that by following his step-by-step instructions, concentrating, and putting forth 100 percent of your effort, you will receive 100 percent of the benefits physically, mentally, and emotionally, regardless of the final position. Trying the right way also means the absence of props, adjustments, and modifications, which are considered crutches in the Bikram tradition; this approach forces students to reach their maximum potential in their *asana* practice of their own accord, without assistance from props, the teacher, or anything else. Bikram yoga teachers rarely give individual feedback; new students just do what they can do according to the instructions given. Most often teachers rely on the "look and see" approach, asking newer students to watch the other students perform the pose during the first round and then try the pose themselves the second time around. Instead of adjusting the pose to compensate for the body's limitations, Choudhury attests that when students attempt wholeheartedly to perform the posture the right way, their bodies will eventually adapt to the poses.

BE PREPARED TO SWEAT

The heat and humidity force the body to sweat out toxins, serving to speed up the natural detoxifying processes while protecting the joints and assisting flexibility. However, the sauna-like atmosphere requires precautions, and you'll want to be prepared for your first Bikram yoga class. Drink plenty of water before, during, and after class; do not eat at least two hours prior to class; wear light, form-fitting clothing (don't be afraid to go skimpy!); and bring a large towel — you're going to need it.

Although billed as a beginner's yoga class, new students are by no means expected to be able to do all the postures in the series (only that they attempt to do them in the right way) or keep up with the pace of class. The extreme heat and conditions of a Bikram yoga class can be quite overwhelming, and students are emphatically encouraged to listen to their bodies and take breaks to sit or lie down on their mats at any point the heat becomes too much. In case you've forgotten, classes are held in 105-degree heat with 40 percent humidity on a lightly carpeted floor, replicating the climate conditions of India. You will begin to sweat within the first five minutes of class and continue to sweat throughout the remainder of the ninety minutes. By the time you're done, every shred of clothing on your body will be drenched in sweat. It's not uncommon to become lightheaded or nauseated during class as a result of dehydration. Feel free to take as many breaks as necessary to sip water and recover (in fact, please do so). The most important thing is that you are there, in class, for the full ninety minutes.

When you first walk into a Bikram yoga class you'll notice that most of those already there are lying flat on their back with their head toward the front mirror. Feel free to lay your mat down in line with the others and take Corpse Pose, relaxing until class begins. Once the teacher enters the room, students will come to stand at the front of their mats, where class begins with the first breathing exercise, Standing Deep Breathing. As you stand with your feet together and fingers interlaced under your chin, the breathing exercise involves slowly inhaling through the nose and exhaling through the mouth in conjunction with tilting the head forward and back while raising and lowering the elbows. Designed to increase lung capacity, bring oxygen to the bloodstream, and awaken every area of the body, the deep breathing helps you relax and focus inwardly, calming and controlling the mind in preparation for the strenuous challenge ahead. The *pranayama* exercise is then followed by twelve standing postures.

There is no flow between positions in Bikram yoga, and you do not need to complete the previous pose before attempting the next. Held for ten to sixty seconds, each pose is performed twice, ending and beginning with feet together at the front of the mat in what is known as neutral position. Once the standing poses are complete, the entire class will lie flat on their back for a two-minute Savasana. The last thirty minutes of class are done on the floor, attempting either seated or supine poses and resting for twenty seconds in Savasana after each posture. Coming up from Corpse Pose requires a sit-up every time, strengthening the abs and realigning the spine for the next seated posture. The twenty-sixth pose and final exercise in the Bikram series is known as "Blowing in Firm." It involves performing Kapalabhati *Pranayama* (Skull Shining Breath) while in Virasana (Hero Pose). The strong Kapalabhati *Pranayama* forces every last bit of carbon dioxide out to make room for fresh oxygen, improves circulation, and strengthens the abdomen muscles and elasticity of the lungs. Class concludes with one last (and much anticipated) Savasana, which some students remain in long after the teacher has exited the room.

THE SECRET OF SAVASANA

Yoga postures twist, squeeze, stretch, and release various muscle groups as well as internal organs, temporarily cutting off blood flow to certain parts of the body. Resting in Savasana between poses allows the entire body to relax and fresh oxygenated blood to rush into the targeted areas for the full physical benefits of each *asana*.

After your first few Bikram yoga classes you will most likely be physically exhausted, which is a good indicator that the body has started the cleansing process. *Hatha* yoga works to remove waste products from all of the organs and glands of the body, which are flushed out through the skin as you sweat (perspiration being the key element of Bikram yoga). As toxins surface, you might feel sick or experience slight skin irritation or both. Don't worry, these symptoms are expected and will normalize after your first several classes. To offset the immense amount of sweating that takes place in one ninety-minute class, Bikram yoga teachers suggest you drink sixty-four to eighty ounces of water in addition to the daily sixty-four to eighty ounces recommended by nutritionists. You may also have a massive headache due to dehydration and the depletion of electrolytes, which can be avoided by taking potassium and salt tablets prior to class. Again, don't worry: It typically takes ten classes to become accustomed to the 105-degree heat. Conversely, you could feel completely euphoric after your first Bikram yoga classes. Students often report feelings of mental clarity and elation after practice. Regardless of the way you feel, even if it's terrible, the best thing to do is to return to class as soon as possible, remembering that once you've established a regular practice your body will adjust to, and even crave, Bikram yoga practice.

The Bikram Series: A Complete Workout

Bikram yoga is above all else effective and efficient. Each posture and breathing exercise in the series serves to address something different in the body; combined, they work every major muscle group, joint, and internal organ, revitalizing and restoring a healthy balance to the body's many systems, including the respiratory, endocrine, digestive, and nervous systems. Within the series, the yoga postures are methodically sequenced so that each pose prepares the body for the next *asana*, warming and stretching the muscles, ligaments, and tendons in the order in which they need to be stretched and never overusing a particular muscle group. The sequence itself focuses on spinal mobility, extension, and strength and is designed to bring the musculoskeletal system back to its natural healthy alignment, safely toning the body, repairing old injuries, and eliminating chronic pain. Although the yoga poses themselves create heat and are designed to change and reshape the body's structure from the inside out, external heat is used in Bikram yoga to warm up the body more quickly. A warm body is a more flexible body, and you may find yourself going deeper into the challenging postures than ever before, which can be advantageous or disadvantageous, depending on whom you ask. Proponents of Bikram and other hot yoga classes claim that the heated room and the resulting increased flexibility lessen the risk of injury, whereas adversaries uphold that the external heat enables students to stretch beyond the healthy limitations of their muscles and ligaments. Just to be cautious: Never force your body into a position. Instead, use the extra warmth of your body to soften and ease deeper into the posture, paying attention to any internal cues that may be warning you to back off.

GET YOUR CARDIO ON

Although there's no flow, and Bikram yoga isn't considered traditional aerobics, the added element of heat provides the cardiovascular benefits of practice. Working to hold each pose for up to a minute regardless of the class environment is going to raise your body temperature; holding yoga postures in 105-degree heat and 40 percent humidity is going to raise your body temperature exponentially. Your heart, your metabolism, and all the systems of your body have to work that much harder to keep your body cool, kicking your cardiovascular system into overdrive. That being said, if you have a medical condition, such as heart disease, high blood pressure, or diabetes, or if you may be pregnant, please consult your doctor before attending your first Bikram yoga class.

Each posture in Bikram yoga is accompanied by a specific breathing technique that is appropriate for that pose. Aside from the first and last *asanas* in the series, which include their own *pranayama* exercises, there are two methods of breathing for the postures. The 80–20 breathing technique is used during standing poses, backbends, and other postures that require oxygen in the lungs to be able to perform with the proper strength. Start by taking a full inhalation, expanding and lifting your rib cage. As you enter the pose, exhale (through your nose) 20 percent of the air that is now in your lungs. Holding the posture, continue to breathe in this manner, inhaling fully and exhaling 20 percent of the air while keeping your lungs 80 percent full. In contrast, the achievement of certain other poses, such as seated forward folds, requires a complete exhalation. After taking a full inhalation, exhale all of the air out of your lungs as you execute the pose. In the beginning you'll probably find either breathing method, or both, difficult to follow. Instead of straining, which Choudhury warns against, take an extra breath or two as needed. With regular practice your lung capacity will expand, and the methods of breathing will become a natural part of your Bikram yoga practice.

With twenty-six postures practiced twice in the same order to nearly the same instructions in every class, Bikram yoga is repetitive. Although this style is considered too boring by some, many students discover that they actually enjoy the repetitious nature of class. For one thing, knowing what's coming next in the series is calming, freeing your mind to focus solely on the present pose; also, revisiting the same yoga postures day after day allows you to become familiar with your weaknesses (the specific aspects of practice that need cultivating), as well as to chart your progress. Within the Bikram method, the only standard of comparison is within your own practice: How do your strength and flexibility, understanding and concentration in a pose compare with the point at which you began? Progress in the system has little to do with doing the twenty-six postures perfectly and more to do with the time, effort, and dedication you give to your yoga practice.

WHERE'S DOWN DOG?

You won't find any inversions (headstands, shoulder stands, handstands, etc.) in Bikram's beginner's yoga class, not even a single Downward-Facing Dog. Believing inversions are too difficult for beginning yoga students, Choudhury chose to leave inverted postures out of his series, incorporating less-advanced poses that provide some of the same benefits.

Raja Yoga: Exercise in Willpower

No matter how fit or experienced you are, Bikram yoga is going to push you beyond your limits, not only physically, but mentally as well. To be able to stay calm, centered, and present in 105-degree heat and 40 percent humidity while you hold challenging standing postures and stretch deeply requires a remarkable will of strength. There is an element of suffering unique to Bikram yoga, and you will be uncomfortable; however, if you make it through an entire class, the feelings of accomplishment are overwhelmingly empowering. Working directly with the body and the mind, the demanding system cultivates the mental faculties of determination, concentration, self-control, faith, and patience.

Therefore, Bikram yoga is considered a combination of *hatha* and *raja* (or royal) yoga. Known as the path of meditation, *raja* yoga is the aspect of the practice that is going to test your willpower, demanding your complete presence in order to perform a pose. The concentration required to follow the step-by-step instructions exactly as they are delivered in class ties the mind to the body. The specific way in which Bikram teachers deliver instructions is meant to keep you completely engaged in the present and immersed in the sequence. The practice itself becomes a ninety-minute meditation: So focused on the task at hand, the mind becomes liberated.

BEYOND SUFFERING

True to classical yoga's philosophy, Bikram yoga uses the body to control the mind by enforcing a very rigid and disciplined practice. As you struggle through the series, the limit of what you believe you're capable of expands, and so also does your perception of who and what you are. You suffer in order to realize you are not your body or your mind; your true Self is much larger, more pervasive, and beyond the limitations and suffering of manifested life. Choudhury attests that by suffering through his yoga class, you will experience an expansion of your entire life.

The method and languaging of the instructions are also designed to bring you into a deep encounter with yourself. Every Bikram yoga studio has at least one mirror (more often many) lining the front wall, and class is done looking at your own reflection. Practicing in front of a mirror, you're able to *see* whether you're doing a pose correctly, whether your legs are straight or bent, the placement of your hips, knees, and shoulders, and so forth. However, being able to look at yourself in this way — not always easy to do, especially when you're sweating and struggling and not wearing a whole lot of clothes — can be a powerfully transformative experience. Standing and looking at your physical body in the mirror, you begin to see beyond the surface and deep inside yourself. The mirror is a tool for self-discovery, the discovery of your true Self. You can, of course, avoid your own reflection or use the mirror to pick on your imperfections, comparing yourself to the woman in the bikini behind you, or you can use the mirror as it is intended: to practice radical self-acceptance. Using the mirror this way, with nowhere to hide and nothing to distract you, you get to practice loving all of yourself for ninety minutes — every wrinkle, every excess fold of skin, every inch of your body from head to toe. Most important, you get to see the real beauty and perfection that reside on the inside. You learn to love yourself and recognize the same beauty in others.

Conclusion

More than any other style on the market, Bikram yoga divides the crowd directly down the middle: People either love it or hate it, often for the same reasons. Those that hate Bikram yoga often don't get it. They hate the heat, the challenge, and the rigidity of the practice. They don't see the point. Those that love the practice, get it. They enjoy the strong discipline and challenge; they even become addicted to the heat and natural high induced by the rush of endorphins and dizzying boosts of oxygen through the body. Devoted students are willing to suffer through "Bikram's torture chamber" four, five, six times a week, because the practice has transformed their health and invigorated their lives. They become oriented toward feeling good and make the necessary lifestyle changes to take better care of themselves and their bodies.

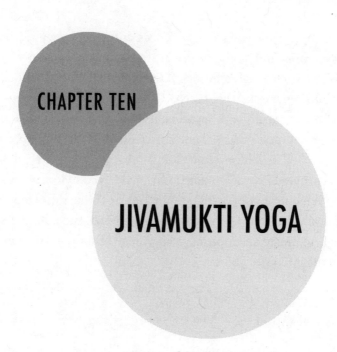

CHAPTER TEN

JIVAMUKTI YOGA

Jivamukti yoga incorporates traditional yoga practices into a modern lifestyle without losing sight of the ancient, universal goal of liberation. We believe that liberation is possible even while living a modern urban lifestyle anywhere in the world. We believe that the ancient teachings and techniques of yoga, as laid out in Patanjali's *Yoga Sutras*, the *Bhagavad Gita*, and the *Hatha Yoga Pradipika*, are as valid and exciting today as they were over five thousand years ago.

— **SHARON GANNON** and **DAVID LIFE**, founders of Jivamukti yoga

Introduction: Ancient Teachings in a Modern Context

Jivamukti yoga is a physically dynamic, intellectually stimulating, and emotionally inspiring practice that is grounded in the universal goal of yoga: enlightenment, or spiritual awareness that leads to the realization of the oneness of being. The method emphasizes the living spiritual tradition of yoga, bringing ancient yogic practices and teachings alive in a contemporary setting and applying the profound wisdom to daily life while fusing old, new, classical, and innovative spiritual and social beliefs and attitudes into a syncretic approach. Classes are in the *vinyasa*-style of practice (linking breath with movement as you flow through a sequence of postures) and incorporate chanting, meditation, *pranayama*, and deep relaxation as well as a heavy injection of philosophy, poetry, music, and devotional prayer. A complete spiritual practice, the style attracts students who are looking for a good workout plus more of what the comprehensive yoga tradition has to offer in ways of emotional, mental, and spiritual well-being, to create an inspiring community of individuals seeking liberation in this lifetime.

LIVING LIBERATION

Jivamukti basically means, "liberation while living." The name is derived from the Sanskrit term *jivanmukti*, which is used to describe the self-realized state of enlightenment. *Jivanmukta* signifies someone who has become liberated from the cycles of *karma* while incarnate. Founders Gannon and Life chose to name their method Jivamukti yoga as a constant reminder to their students that the ultimate aim of practicing yoga is spiritual enlightenment and awareness.

Emerging from one of New York City's most popular yoga studios, Jivamukti yoga was created and founded by David Life and Sharon Gannon in 1984. Both students of Sri K. Pattabhi Jois, they combined their studies of Ashtanga yoga with spiritual teachings they received from their other two gurus, Swami Nirmalananda and Sri Brahmananda Sarasvati, as well as their own talents and ventures as artists, performers, and musicians, to develop their innovative approach to yoga. Their core philosophy — enlightenment through compassion for all beings — is reflected in Jivamukti yoga's main teachings, which revolve around animal rights, vegetarianism/veganism, environmentalism, and social activism, as well as in the style's passionate embrace of the original meaning of the Sanskrit term *asana* as "seat," expanded to mean "connection or relationship to the earth" (implying all living things). Therefore, the *asana* practice, which the method is based upon, isn't as much about the physical yoga postures and maintaining a healthy, fit body as it is about every relationship you have, on and off the mat. Ultimately, the practice of *asana* (that is, showing compassion and kindness for all beings) leads to the dissolution of the sense of otherness, or separateness, and the experience of union with divine consciousness, which is to say enlightenment.

Gannon and Life met their first guru, Swami Nirmalananda, on a trip to India in 1986. Living in his solitary *ashram* hidden deep in the forest in southern India, Swami Nirmalananda was a vegan, naturalist, and self-proclaimed anarchist (known as the "anarchist swami") who wrote hundreds of letters to international leaders pleading for world peace and spreading his message of *ahimsa*, do no harm, worldwide. Although Gannon and Life were already passionate about animal rights and active members of PETA prior to meeting their first guru, Nirmalananda's teachings and personal practice affirmed for them that political activism plays an essential role on the spiritual path. The swami also taught them Jivamukti yoga's core *mantra*: *lokah samastah sukhino bhavantu*, translated to mean "May all beings, everywhere, be happy and free." The extended interpretation by Gannon, "May all living beings, everywhere, be happy and free, and may the thoughts, words and actions of my own life contribute to that happiness and to that freedom for all," is repeated in every class or gathering.

Two years later on a subsequent trip to India, the partners met their second guru, Sri K. Pattabhi Jois. Unlike Swami Nirmalananda, who was an ascetic renunciant and a *mauni* (someone who practices silence, which Nirmalananda did for eleven years), Jois was a householder with a wife and family, teaching his Ashtanga-vinyasa yoga to the public. Jois showed Gannon and Life that it is possible, and necessary, to remain active in this world while walking the yogic path, and he expounded the ethical and philosophical principles of classical yoga to them. Paying homage to Jois, Gannon and Life adopted his rigorous *vinyasa* sequence as the foundation for Jivamukti yoga's *asana* practice. Following Jois's teachings, they also integrated the study of yogic texts into their *hatha* yoga classes, encouraging students to read the Yoga Sutras of Patanjali and continually emphasizing the importance of keeping the highest aspirations of yoga in mind while practicing.

GURU BLESSINGS

Having spent years studying with their various gurus, Gannon and Life exhibit great respect, gratitude, and devotion to their teachings, which undoubtedly helped shape the development of Jivamukti yoga. Honoring the teacher-disciple tradition of yoga, they received individual blessings from each of their gurus to incorporate the guru's practices and teachings into the Jivamukti method.

The two spiritual seekers met their third guru, Sri Brahmananda Sarasvati, in 1995 at his Ananda Ashram in Monroe, New York. Brahmananda Sarasvati was a highly educated swami with an extensive background in both Eastern and Western medicine, and for a number of years he practiced medicine as Dr. Ramamurti Mishra in India and the United States before taking *sannyas* (vows of renunciation). Also a prolific writer and Sanskrit scholar, he is the author of *Fundamentals of Yoga: The Textbook of Yoga Psychology* (a commentary on the Yoga Sutras) and *Self Analysis and Self Knowledge*. Brahmananda dedicated his life to the synthesis of Eastern and Western science, philosophy, and culture, founding the Yoga Society of New York in 1958 and the Ananda Ashram six years later, where his teachings continue to be taught and followed by devotees. His eternal message — "You are not the body and mind, although you have a body and mind. You are the Self," which is beyond the body and mind — greatly influenced Gannon and Life's spiritual path and thus the development of Jivamukti yoga. The guru also stressed the importance of meditation and Sanskrit study, which is emphasized in the Jivamukti method, as well as in the practice of *nada* yoga (the yoga of sound), which is one of the method's five fundamental tenets.

Gannon and Life have coauthored three books: *Jivamukti Yoga: Practices for Liberating Body and Soul* (2002); *The Art of Yoga* (2002); and *Yoga*

Assists (2013). Their Jivamukti Yoga School in New York City is among the most noted and influential in the country. Credited by *Vanity Fair* with "making yoga cool and hip," the innovative founders have established a method of teaching yoga as spiritual practice in a modern context, expounding the teachings of their gurus and illuminating the deep, esoteric wisdom of the yoga tradition through their profound creativity and ability to adapt the language of the teachings without "dumbing down" the concepts.

The Gist: One Method, a Variety of Classes

A Jivamukti yoga class is equal parts physical, educational, and inspirational, designed to invigorate and energize students while taking them on a spiritual journey of self-discovery. Jivamukti teachers are generally very friendly, kind, and insightful and are often artists, musicians, or other types of performers in their own right. At the very least, they are unique self-expressionists who are encouraged to interpret and share yoga's ancient teachings in their own creative ways. On that note, each class has a theme, usually drawn from the Focus of the Month (written by either Gannon or Life), which is explored through scriptures, philosophical concepts, music, chanting, meditation, breathing exercises, and even the sequence of *asanas* itself. Having a theme, or focus, for class produces context and gives students an attitudinal direction for their practice, creating meaning and making class personally relevant. Having a monthly focus allows Jivamukti students to hear and experience the same profound concept, such as sacred geometry, the *chakra* system, or death, in a variety of ways and from different perspectives.

There are six types of classes in the Jivamukti yoga method. If you're newer to *asana* practice or if you haven't been practicing with much alignment, the Jivamukti basic class is the best place to begin. Each class is part of a four-week fundamentals course covering the main groups of *asanas*: standing poses (week one), forward bending poses (week two), backward bending poses (week three), and inverted postures (week four). Teachers are given a set curriculum for the course, teaching the *asanas* in the specified sequence while explaining in detail how to do each pose, including how to use props to modify the postures. For example, during the first week of every month, only standing poses will be taught in Jivamukti basic classes and in the same order every time. Rather than holding each pose for an extended length of time, you'll be given the opportunity to do each pose at least twice. Every basic class includes a ten-minute Savasana as the teacher guides you to relax each body part in succession from feet to forehead.

RAISING THE BAR

Jivamukti yoga is known for setting high teacher-training standards, requiring teachers to complete a month-long residential program totaling three hundred hours, compared with the two hundred hours required for almost all other styles of yoga. Teachers who complete the three-hundred-hour training leave feeling empowered and confident and are knowledgeable in all aspects of Jivamukti yoga, including how to incorporate the physical, psychological, spiritual, and mystic components of the yoga tradition into their daily lives as well as how to teach students to do the same. Once teachers have completed training at the three-hundred-hour level, they may choose to enter the system's apprenticeship program for an additional five hundred hours of teacher training (i.e., for eight hundred hours in total). Advanced certifications are also offered, allowing teachers who qualify to become mentors, operate their own Jivamukti yoga center, serve on review boards, and so forth.

A different theme is explored each week along with the alignment and structure of the group of poses, which are also set: Week one, standing *asanas* are about grounding, reflecting your willingness to be here and connect to the earth; week two, forward bending turns you inward, back into your past, allowing you to release emotions stored in the hamstrings, hips, and spine; week three, backbends open the thighs, abdomen, chest, and throat, releasing fears and trapped emotions related to those areas of the body, allowing you to move forward in your life and practice; and week four emphasizes "putting it all together," introducing students to inversions as well as meditation and integrating the physical, mental, emotional, and spiritual layers of self. Students who are new to Jivamukti yoga are encouraged to enroll in the entire four-week course, but anyone can drop in for a basic class at any time during the month.

The style's beginner *vinyasa* class provides the perfect transition between basic classes and the style's more rigorous and fast-paced flow practices. Class begins with the chanting of Jivamukti's core *mantra* to set the intention, followed by an explanation of *vinyasa*, the three components of *vinyasa* (*asana*, breath, and intention), and instructions on the *ujjayi* breathing technique. Teaching the basic fundamentals of a *vinyasa* practice, beginner *vinyasa* classes switch the focus from the alignment of the *asanas* to the breath. Moving slowly, students learn how to safely and smoothly transition in and out of the *asanas* while synchronizing their breath with the movements, as well as how to breathe and count their breaths while holding postures. The learning environment is very relaxed; students are encouraged to freely explore the deeper aspects of *vinyasa* practice, while the teacher helps them understand how to move with their inhalations and exhalations, calling out transitions to keep the breathing pace steady. This is the one Jivamukti yoga class in which music may not be played, since the teacher talks almost continuously.

DEFINING *VINYASA*

Within the Jivamukti method, *vinyasa* (*vi* meaning "sequence" and *nyasa* meaning "to place in a special way") is the practice of aligning both your breath and your intention with movement as you flow through the series of *asanas*. Without intention, *asana* practice doesn't lead to a state of spiritual awareness. Students are encouraged to remember the selfless intention set forth in the opening *mantra*: "to contribute to the happiness and freedom of others." Consciously aligning all three — breath, movement, and intention — calms and focuses the mind in the direction of yoga: union or unity with all.

For the full, magical Jivamukti yoga experience, attend an open class and prepare to be transformed. This is where the relevance of the classical yoga teachings is really driven home, and Jivamukti teachers shine as creative individuals. Students are seamlessly led through a flowing *vinyasa* sequence of postures accompanied by an eclectic sound track of exuberant music, such as ragas, reggae, global trance, hip-hop, indie rock, classical music, blues, and pop. Every Jivamukti open class incorporates fourteen points (see sidebar on page 161). The exact sequence itself is creatively designed by the teacher. Students are invited to work at their own pace, with the teacher giving beginner, intermediate, and advanced *asana* options (although without many detailed how-to descriptions) and offering skillful hands-on assistance while paying close attention to the correct alignment and form of the poses. Throughout class you will be gently reminded of the intention you set at the beginning of the practice and prompted to be aware of your breath.

HANDS-ON APPROACH

You can expect to be touched in an open class; Jivamukti yoga teachers are known for their effective hands-on adjustments and are quite adept at the art of teaching with touch. However, if you're at all uncomfortable receiving manual adjustments or just don't like being touched, let the teacher know, and he or she will honor that.

Jivamukti's signature "spiritual warrior" class is designed for busy people who are interested in a robust *asana* workout but don't have much time to devote to their daily yoga practice. In one hour, students are led through a brisk *vinyasa* flow sequence while the teacher calls out the *asanas*, provides breath count, and keeps the pace moving, giving minimal instructions on how to do the postures. Class begins with Jivamukti's standardized warm-up series, dubbed the "Magic Ten" (ten simple exercises that can be done in about ten minutes), immediately followed by intention setting. Standing at the front of your mat, you'll be invited first to think of someone you love, someone who is challenging you, or someone who is suffering and then to dedicate your practice to that person —

offering your practice to something outside yourself. Together, the class will then chant: *om om om shantih shantih shantih hari om*, which will be repeated at the end of practice as well.

The well-rounded class sequence is set, beginning with three rounds of traditional ashtanga Surya Namaskar A's (Sun Salutations), followed by one round of Jivamukti's version of Surya Namaskar, leading directly into standing poses, backbends, forward bends, twists, and inversions, ending with a five-minute silent meditation and Savasana. Designed to be invigorating yet simultaneously grounding, the fixed sequence allows students to learn and memorize the *asanas* quickly while building a steady, consistent *sadhana* (or spiritual) practice and is best for intermediate and advanced students.

THE FOURTEEN POINTS COVERED IN A JIVAMUKTI OPEN CLASS

1. Surya Namaskar
2. Side bend, such as Trikonasana
3. Twist: Ardha Matsyendrasana (Half Lord of the Fishes Pose) or Parvritta Parsvakonasana (Revolved Side Angle Pose)

Backbends, including

4. Bhujangasana (Cobra Pose) or Shalabhasana (Locust Pose)
5. Dhanurasana (Bow Pose), Ustrasana (Camel Pose), or Rabbit Pose
6. Urdhva Dhanurasana (Wheel Pose)

7. Paschimottanasana (Seated Forward Bend)
8. Purvottanasana (Upward Plank), Tabletop, or Half-Wheel
9. Supta Baddha Konasana (Reclining Bound Angle Pose) or Matsyasana (Fish Pose)

Inversions, including

10. Adho Mukha Vriksasana (Handstand), Shirsasana (Headstand), or Pincha Mayurasana (Forearm Stand)
11. Sarvangasana (Shoulder Stand) and Halasana (Plow Pose), or Viparita Karani (Legs-up-the-Wall)

12. Savasana
13. Meditation
14. Spiritual teachings

Completely unique to the Jivamukti yoga system, in-class privates (or ICPs) are offered, which involve a private teacher accompanying you to a class (the most popular being an open class). Throughout the entire class, the teacher assists your practice with hands-on adjustments, safely guiding you through the *asanas* with correct alignment and making sure you understand all of the other spiritual components of class. Jivamukti teachers suggest having one or two ICPs a year to keep reviewing and refreshing your alignment in the postures. ICPs are also ideal for students who have injuries and are seeking to use their yoga practice to help recover and heal. The bonus: a special deep relaxation massage during Savasana.

Meditation classes are held at least once a week at Jivamukti yoga centers, offering students a more complete introduction and experience of seated meditation than are presented in the other types of Jivamukti yoga classes. The method uses a *mantra* form of meditation practice, following three simple instructions: choose a comfortable seat, be still, and focus. To clear the energy in the atmosphere, class begins with a Sanskrit chant followed by specific meditation instructions given by the teacher. The *mantra* "let go" provides the focus. Silently repeating "let" on the inhalation and "go" on the exhalation, students are encouraged to allow their breath to flow freely through the body as well as thoughts through the mind, without trying to control or manipulate either. With the suggestion of letting go (of control as well as any thoughts that arise or sensations felt in the body) and the sustained focus required to align the *mantra* with the breath, students begin to let go of their identification with the body and the mind, allowing self-realization to arise spontaneously. After about twenty minutes of seated, silent meditation, class concludes with a Q&A session led by the teacher and then a closing prayer.

Core Philosophy:
"Enlightenment through Compassion for All Beings"

Central to the practice of Jivamukti yoga is the radical understanding and embrace of *ahimsa* (the Sanskrit term for nonviolence or restraint from harming others), emphasizing a profound respect and care for all living beings that includes the practice of ethical vegetarianism or veganism and the protection of animal rights. Gannon and Life, who have been criticized for being too political — their promotion of a vegetarian lifestyle considered too extreme for a yoga school — founded the Jivamukti method on the belief that in order to coexist in harmony, every individual must take responsibility for his or her part in the collective creation of our communities and living environments. They maintain that caring for and helping others are not only fundamental aspects of any spiritual practice but also the best ways to uplift your own life and spirit, and that avoiding the exploitation of animals for experimentation or entertainment or the use of animal products, whether for food, clothes, or accessories such as furniture, is "the single greatest act" anyone can do for the betterment of others and the world at large. On a mission to dismantle our present-day culture, which Gannon asserts is "based on the old paradigm...which tells us that 'the earth belongs to us' and exists for us to exploit," through their teachings they emphasize the importance of living the practice of nonviolence or doing no harm rather than merely conceptualizing *ahimsa* in the classroom.

ETHICAL PRECEPTS OF YOGA

Ahimsa is one of the five *yamas* (or restrictions) of classical yoga. While the aim of Patanjali's eight-limbed yoga is to experience enlightenment, if you still perceive others as being separate from you, then the *yamas* advise that you should not harm others, lie to them, steal from them, sexually exploit them, or be greedy, any of which leads directly away from the realization that we are all united and interconnected.

The Jivamukti yoga method emphasizes the exploration of the true, applicable, and physical meaning of the Sanskrit term *asana*, which is taken to mean "relationship" and is understood as "our relationship to the earth," dissolving the illusion of separateness through kindness, compassion, and restraint from causing harm. Gannon proposes, "What could be more physical than what we eat, where we live, and who we live with?"

In addition to urging the practice of vegetarianism or veganism and the protection of animal rights, the founders heavily advocate social activism and environmentalism, claiming that they (and their school of yoga) can't help but be political. Because they believe that living beings are not separate but rather united in one spirit, they assert that anything and everything that one person does affects the whole. Gannon and Life proclaim that to be conscious of how your choices and actions affect others, the environment, and every living organism on earth *is* to be politically active. They warn their students not to remain encapsulated in their little "yoga bubble," encouraging them instead to care about their communities and positively contribute to the welfare and happiness of others.

Five Tenets

The method's core philosophy (that our relationship to the earth is the means to attaining enlightenment in this lifetime) is reflected in Jivamukti's five tenets: *ahimsa* (compassion), *dhyana* (meditation), *bhakti* (devotion), *nada* (sound), and *shastra* (scripture). These five elements, embodied by all of the style's teachers, are assimilated into the practices, instructions, interactions, and even environment at Jivamukti yoga centers, which incorporate eco-friendly materials and adhere to incredibly high "green" standards.

JIVAMUKTI OPEN CLASS

While all five elements — *ahimsa, dhyana, bhakti, nada,* and *shashtra* — form the foundation of every Jivamukti yoga class, they are specifically integrated into a unified practice in the system's open classes. Whether or not the specific terms are used or explicitly covered, each of the five tenets must be clearly identifiable in open classes, and teachers must incorporate each principal element into their class plan, allowing them to inform their teaching style. This way, students begin to understand that the five precepts are an integral part of spiritual practice and not separate from *asana* practice.

Gannon and Life maintain that meditation, both its study and its practice, is a necessary component of any spiritual practice and is crucial in the quest for spiritual attainment — that without meditation there's "no point in practicing *asanas*." That being said, teachers continually remind students to stay present and remain focused throughout the practice, and every Jivamukti yoga class includes at least a five-minute seated meditation. As mentioned previously, each class also has a theme, serving to promote the educational aspects of yoga practice. *Shastra* refers to the study of ancient Indian scriptures. Jivamukti yoga teachers draw from the four main yogic texts: the Yoga Sutras of Patanjali, the Hatha-Yoga-Pradipika, the Bhagavad Gita, and the Upanishads, which students are encouraged to study as well, in addition to the Sanskrit alphabet and language.

Bhakti, meaning "devotion to God," is expressed through chanting, praying, setting an intention, and acknowledging that Self-realization is the highest aspiration of practicing yoga. Jivamukti yoga seeks to develop interfaith understanding and tolerance for all religions, not caring which form of the Divine you choose as the target of your devotion, just that you devote yourself, and your practice, to something bigger than yourself. Blending Eastern and Western religious and spiritual traditions, images of Jesus, Buddha, Shiva, and Krishna, as well as Gandhi, Martin Luther King Jr., Ingrid Newkirk, and other moral authorities adorn the walls of most Jivamukti yoga centers, and candlelit altars and burning incense help enhance the devotional ambience. Along with the chanting of *mantras*, Jivamukti yoga emphasizes the repetition of the names of God, most notably "Hari Om," as an important part of the yoga practice, which brings us to the last tenet: *nada*. Chanting, which integrates scriptural study with *bhakti* practice, is also an aspect of *nada* yoga, or the yoga of sound.

Nada yoga centers on deep inner listening for the unstruck, or silent, sound — *om*, as the primordial vibration of the entire universe. However, one's ability to hear and listen must be developed first. Jivamukti yoga facilitates this development by incorporating elevated music, the spoken word, *kirtan* (call-and-response chanting), and silence into the *asana* practice, along with the verbal instructions given by the teacher.

In class teachers play an assorted array of music, from Krishna Das and Ravi Shankar to Moby and the Beatles, intentionally chosen to support the theme of practice and to evoke feelings of devotion while cultivating students' ability to listen for the subtle vibration of *om*.

KIRTAN CONCERTS

Kirtan involves the devotional chanting of Sanskrit *mantras* sung in a group, led by a *kirtan* musician, and usually accompanied by a harmonium, drums, and other classical Indian instruments. Concerts are festive events during which everyone in the crowd joins in, chanting, clapping, swaying, and dancing along to the rhythmic chanting. The songs range from ten to thirty minutes long, and each is followed by a period of silence to allow the effects of the *mantras* to sink in. Originally introduced by Krishna Das, the *kirtan* movement has become quite popular in recent years — the Jivamukti Yoga Center in New York being one of the premiere *kirtan* concert venues. Other big names in the kirtan world include Jai Uttal, Deva Premal, Wah!, and Dave Stringer.

Conclusion

Integrating scriptural study, meditation, sound, and devotional elements into the practice of *asana* and relaxation, Jivamukti yoga presents a complete spiritual path of living liberation. Students are attracted to the profound insight and spiritual relevance imparted in Jivamukti yoga classes. They are spiritual seekers, as well as activists for social and animal rights and committed to awakening and living more consciously. Jivamukti teachers, like the style's founders, aren't subtle about their beliefs and values, in accordance with the method's fundamental precepts, attracting like-minded individuals and creating a community of people who really care about one another and the world at large.

CHAPTER ELEVEN

BEST OF THE REST

The vibrant American yoga scene is in continual flux, pulsating with new styles and teachers, contemporary innovations and interpretations, and a myriad of students and communities. Aside from the widely known systems depicted in the previous chapters, there are traditional guru-based styles that have been around since the 1970s and never reached mainstream popularity, some that were once thriving and have since faded into the background, and still others being born and moving into the spotlight every year. Listing and describing all of the yoga systems and styles on the market today, many of which don't fit neatly into a cubbyhole, would be nearly impossible. In this chapter you will find ten more styles, giving you a well-rounded view of the yoga being practiced in the West. Still others are not discussed here, such as Rod Stryker's Para yoga, Cindi Lee's Om yoga, Kali Ray's TriYoga, and Jill Miller's Yoga Tune-Up, not to mention the innumerable types of *vinyasa* flow classes.

Sivananda Yoga: Five Principles of Yoga

A very traditional form of yoga, Sivananda yoga aims to cultivate the health and vitality of the body and mind, naturally leading to spiritual evolution. The method revolves around five main principles: proper exercise (*asana*), proper breathing (*pranayama*), proper relaxation (Savasana), proper diet (vegetarianism), and positive thinking (Vedanta) and meditation (*dhyana*). Easy to learn, the training system is standardized into a basic class structure that follows a set combination of breathing exercises, Sun Salutations (Surya Namaskar), and twelve yoga postures with frequent relaxation between poses. The method includes classes at the beginning, intermediate, and advanced levels, allowing for variations of the twelve classic postures and even a few extra *asanas*, depending on the level of the students.

Developed by Swami Vishnu-devananda, who spent ten years in intensive training in all aspects of the yoga tradition at the original Sivananda *ashram*, in India, the traditional method is named after the teachings of his guru, Swami Sivananda. In 1957, Swami Vishnu-devananda arrived in the West, sent by Sivananda to spread the teachings of yoga and Vedanta, and two years later established the first Sivananda Yoga Vedanta Centre, in Montreal, Canada, as well as the International Sivananda Yoga Vedanta Centers, which together serve as a nonprofit organization dedicated to preserving and imparting the authentic teachings of the yoga tradition. Today there are nearly sixty Sivananda locations worldwide, including nine *ashrams* and nineteen yoga centers, as well as a number of affiliate centers. It was Swami Vishnu-devananda who summarized the vast and ancient teachings of yoga into five easy-to-understand principles, giving specific methods for developing and maintaining physical, emotional, and mental health, as well as spiritual growth, for the purpose of incorporating them into one's daily life and practice.

TRUE WORLD ORDER

Along with the International Sivananda Yoga Vedanta Centers, Swami Vishnu-devananda established the True World Order (TWO) to train "future leaders and responsible citizens of the world in yogic disciplines." He was the first to create a yoga teacher-training program in the West. Seeking to impart the skills of personal discipline and daily practice, he based the training program on the ancient Gurukul training system, which mandates that the teachings and wisdom of yoga be integrated into the daily life of sincere aspirants. In the past three decades TWO has trained over twenty-six thousand yoga professionals.

Along with Sivananda yoga's five universal principles, the system seeks to integrate the four main paths of yoga — *karma* (the path of action), *bhakti* (the path of devotion), *raja* (the path of concentration and meditation), and *jnana* (the path of knowledge or wisdom) — similar to the goal of Integral yoga, founded by Sri Swami Satchidananda. Satchidananda and Vishnu-devananda were both close disciples of Swami Sivananda, arriving in the United States within a decade of each other. Recognizing that each individual identifies with his or her body, heart, and mind, Swami Sivananda taught that a well-balanced *sadhana* (personal spiritual discipline) must include aspects of each of the four paths. Different yogas or components of the various yogic paths can be emphasized at different times, depending on a person's temperament and interests, with all paths ultimately leading to the same goal of spiritual attainment. Swami Sivananda's integrated approach became known as the "Yoga of Synthesis."

Every Sivananda yoga class begins and ends in Savasana, either preceding or following the opening and closing prayer in the form of *mantras*. Class itself tends to be more slowly paced, with an internal, meditative focus. Each of the twelve *asanas* is held for a designated length of time, and a full, yogic breath is emphasized, as opposed to the more powerful, stimulating *ujjayi* breath used in more aerobic styles of yoga. The traditional yoga postures not only increase strength, flexibility, and circulation, releasing deeply stored tension in the body, but also align and open the various *chakras*, or energy centers, of the body. The specific order of the yoga poses is designed to systematically move every major muscle and joint in the body, as well as the spine, bringing the entire body back into balance while increasing the flow of *prana* (life-force energy) through the *chakras* and the subtle body. The practice of deep breathing calms and focuses the mind, and the deep relaxation that is built into every class helps relieve symptoms of stress and rejuvenates the nervous system. In the end, Sivananda yoga promotes a yogic lifestyle, applying the teachings to daily life, in which a proper yogic diet is of the utmost importance.

PROPER YOGIC DIET

According to the Sivananda tradition, an integral aspect of the yogic lifestyle is a proper yogic diet, which is lactovegetarian and consists of simple, pure, natural foods that are rich in nutrients and easy to digest. Furthermore, because what we eat affects our entire state, not just the physical body but mental and emotional states as well, a proper yogic diet avoids overstimulating foods and substances, such as garlic, onions, and coffee.

Ananda Yoga: Experience Your Bliss

A spiritually oriented approach to *hatha* yoga, Ananda yoga emphasizes the inner aspects of the practice, that is, paying close attention to the currents of energy through the body and the fluctuations, or states, of the mind as they arise throughout practice. The system was derived from the teachings of Paramahansa Yogananda, who founded the Self-Realization Fellowship, wrote *Autobiography of a Yogi*, and introduced the path of *kriya* yoga to the West, and it was systematized by his close and direct disciple, Swami Kriyananda, founder of Ananda yoga. Yogananda taught that a single blissful consciousness, known as Satchidananda, underlies all existence (the one truth uniting all the world's great religions) and is both infinite and eternal. With this fundamental belief, the Ananda yoga method aims to raise individual consciousness in order for Self-realization to occur — the process of recognizing yourself as a manifestation of the one supreme consciousness that pervades everything (variously called the Divine, God, Allah, Shiva, Buddha-nature, and so forth) — which is achieved mainly by embracing inner silence and meditation.

KRIYA YOGA

Described by Yogananda in his *Autobiography of a Yogi*, *kriya* yoga is an advanced *raja* yoga technique (*raja* yoga being the royal path of Patanjali's eight-limbed yoga) designed to accelerate spiritual evolution. After a year of preparation and practice, using basic meditation techniques outlined by Yogananda, students are initiated into the technique of *kriya* yoga. Once initiated, they accept Yogananda's teachings, also accepting him as their guru and thus becoming his disciples.

An inwardly directed practice, Ananda yoga includes *asana*, emphasizing alignment, safety, and modification of the postures; *pranayama*; energy-control techniques; classical meditation; and applied yoga philosophy. The *asana* practice is considered gentle for beginners but becomes increasingly challenging with experience and dedication, though never aggressive or aerobic. Students are continually encouraged to remain as relaxed as possible, even when the pose requires effort, maintaining an internal awareness the entire class. Each yoga posture is paired with an affirmation silently repeated while in the pose, reinforcing the inherent effects the yoga postures have on our consciousness. With this uplifting practice, students are guided to explore their own spirituality through the *asanas*, which are not separate from the spiritual path of yoga but are simply the third limb of *raja* yoga.

Unique to Ananda yoga are the system's Energization Exercises, developed by Yogananda to help students awaken, increase, and harness *prana* (life-force energy) in the body. A series of thirty-nine energy-control techniques, the Energization Exercises focus on "drawing the cosmic energy into the body through the medulla oblongata by the power of will." The medulla oblongata is the lowest portion of the brain stem and is where the spinal cord merges with the brain. For external reference, it's most identifiable by the occipital bone, which you can feel at the base of the skull and through which the spinal column passes to connect to the brainstem. Long thought of by yogis as the "portal through which the energy enters the body," the medulla oblongata is often referred to as "the mouth of God." Completing the thirty-nine Energization Exercises, which take about ten to twelve minutes to do once you are familiar with the routine, not only increases your life-force energy but also releases any held bodily tension in preparation for longer, seated meditation (the primary practice for attaining god-consciousness).

DOUBLE BREATHING

Yogananda taught a special breathing technique, called "double breathing," which accompanies the Energization Exercises. This technique is fairly simple to do; you begin by taking a quick, short inhalation through the nose and mouth, directly followed by a longer, fuller inhalation. Then you immediately exhale in the same manner: one short exhalation followed by a longer exhalation, making the sound *huh huhhhhhhh* as you breathe out of your mouth and nose.

Viniyoga: Individualized Approach

Viniyoga is all about adaptation and the appropriate application of yogic teachings and practices according to each person's needs, ability, and interests. The method is founded on the traditional guru-disciple model, in which highly knowledgeable and skilled teachers work one-on-one with each student to create a personalized yoga program based on the individual's health, age, and physical conditions and limitations, including past and current injuries, as well as personal potential and intention for practicing. Whether your aim is physical well-being, emotional balance, spiritual attunement, or any combination of these, Viniyoga is designed to teach you how to begin from wherever you are today, giving you the tools necessary to progress toward your individual goals.

INTENTION IS KEY

Yoga is the practice of an intention. Viniyoga encourages students to become very clear about their intention(s) for practicing, whether it be to release tension in the neck and shoulders, strengthen the core, develop confidence, reduce stress, evolve spiritually, or anything else that is appropriate. The clearer and more specific your intention is, the more personalized your yoga program can be — in choosing the specific elements and applications that support your purpose for practicing — and the greater your chances are of realizing your goals.

Gary Kraftsow, director and senior teacher of the American Viniyoga Institute, evolved this individualized approach to yoga from the teachings transmitted by Sri T. Krishnamacharya and his son T. K. V. Desikachar. Kraftsow began his studies with Desikachar in 1974, spending years at a time in India, and has been teaching yoga for health, healing, and personal development for over thirty years in the States and abroad. Upon receiving his master's degree in psychology and religion from the University of California at Santa Barbara, Kraftsow opened the Maui School of Yoga Therapy in 1983, received a Viniyoga special diploma from the Viniyoga International in Paris, in 1988, and in 1999 established the American Viniyoga Institute, which remains dedicated to the authentic transmission of the teachings in his lineage. One of the leading yoga therapists in the United States, Kraftsow travels extensively, giving lectures, workshops, and trainings, and is the author of two published books, *Yoga for Wellness* (1999) and *Yoga for Transformation* (2002), as well as two educational DVDs. He also serves as a yoga research consultant and has developed protocol for two successful National Institutes of Health studies: Evaluating Yoga for Chronic Low Back Pain and Yoga Therapy for Generalized Anxiety.

The Sanskrit term *viniyoga* actually implies differentiation, adaptation, and appropriate application. Drawing from the vast teachings of yoga, including *asana*, *pranayama*, chanting, meditation, personal rituals, and scriptural study, Viniyoga teachers adapt the various means and methods of practice as needed by each individual to foster a greater sense of well-being overall and to support their intention for practicing. The method emphasizes the principles of breath as the main movement in *asana* (altering the breathing pattern while in a pose to generate different therapeutic effects), the biomechanics of the yoga poses, safe sequencing, and function over form, again, adapting the forms of the postures to meet the needs of the individual to achieve various results. Class is a combination of dynamic movements and static holds, maintaining the alignment of poses for a consistent number of breaths with brief periods of rest in between. Viniyoga is also big on repetition in moving in and out of the postures, warming up the body, increasing circulation to targeted areas, and triggering neuromuscular repatterning: The scientific method is designed to replace dysfunctional movement patterns with more functional ones that don't place as much stress on your structure.

Ultimately, the individualized approach is meant to offer students insight into their own nature, initiating a process of self-discovery and personal transformation that is unique to each of them. Viniyoga lays the foundation for the more profound yoga practices in case you desire to deepen your spiritual commitment, though it's not required. Conscious integration of breath and body is an integral component of the method, as is *pranayama*. In addition to preparing and training students for seated meditation, Viniyoga teaches them to be present through continual breath awareness, which calms the mind, balances the nervous system, and relieves stress.

Svaroopa Yoga: Open to Your Own Divinity

Svaroopa yoga promises to bring you into "the bliss of your own being." The method is based on spinal decompression, which Svaroopa calls core release, and is designed to release the deeply held tension in the muscles attached to the spine, opening you up to the experience of your own divinity. A less active style of yoga than others, completely accessible to everyone regardless of his or her physical condition, age, or ability, Svaroopa yoga uses the precise angles and alignment of specific yoga postures to open the spine, beginning at the tailbone and progressing up through each spinal region. With the support of blankets, blocks, and other yoga props, students fully rest into the angles of each pose for a period of time, allowing the core muscles along the spine to relax and the vertebrae to decompress. The effect is healing and transformative, promoting deep relaxation and stress relief that are inherent to the release of your core muscles, while also alleviating back pain as well as shoulder and neck tension.

ABIDE IN YOUR OWN BLISS

In Patanjali's Yoga Sutras, the term *svaroopa* is used to denote the inner experience of pure consciousness. Sutra 1.3 (*tada drashtuh svarupe avasthanam*) translates as "then the seer abides in its own nature." *Svaroopa* means "own form" (*sva* meaning "self" and *roopa* meaning "form"), which is consciousness itself and is loosely translated as "to know yourself at the deepest level of your being," which Svaroopa yoga describes as a state of bliss.

Developed by Swami Nirmalananda Saraswati, who received *shakti-pat-deeksha* (initiation) from Swami Muktananda (head of the Siddha yoga path at the time) in 1976, Svaroopa yoga is designed to give students the experience of "opening from the inside out," known as "core opening." *Shaktipat* is the transmission of energy from a spiritual master that awakens the seeker's own inherent creative power within, known as *kundalini-shakti*, placing him or her on the path of spiritual evolution. The initiation is often described as the "descent of grace," grace being both a state, as in grace filled, and the driving force of conscious awakening, as in grace fueled. (You'll notice that styles of yoga connected to the Siddha yoga lineage refer to grace, especially opening to the flow of grace, as one of their main principles, such as in Svaroopa and Anusara yoga.) After receiving *shaktipat* from Muktananda, Swami Nirmalananda (formerly known as Rama Berch) sold her business and moved her family into the Siddha yoga *ashram* in upstate New York, where she served as part of the management team and taught *asana* classes. Living in the *ashram* allowed her to fully immerse herself in Muktananda's teachings, which laid the foundation for the birth of Svaroopa yoga.

Teaching *hatha* yoga in the *ashram*, she noticed that the students were attempting to impose the positions of the *asanas* upon their bodies, performing the poses from an external point of reference rather than allowing the postures to unfold from within. Frustrated, she began experimenting with different ways of guiding her students into the deeper experience of the *asanas*, eventually designing specific protocols that allow students to have the inner experience of core opening. Swami Nirmalananda has always said that Svaroopa yoga was and is "all a function of grace," maintaining that the poses, precise alignment, and method of resting into the angles of the postures — the entire process of Svaroopa yoga — spontaneously came to her in meditation as a result of receiving *shaktipat* from Muktananda. She describes her teaching methodology as "a cosmic download," given to her by her guru. "He gave it to me in one instant, whole and complete, but it took me fifteen years to figure out what I got." The specific protocols and process of Svaroopa yoga were created by Swami Nirmalananda to give students the same cosmic download she received from her guru, guiding them into their own source of bliss, into their Selves, so that they may experience their own divinity.

SWAMI NIRMALANANDA SARASWATI

Along with trademarking Svaroopa yoga at the urging of her students, Swami Nirmalananda Saraswati founded the Master Yoga Academy and the Svaroopa Vidya Ashram. She also developed and directed the yoga program for Deepak Chopra's Center for Wellbeing, in Carlsbad, California. Initiated into the ancient order of Saraswati monks in 2009, Nirmalananda now dons the traditional orange robes and lives her life dedicated to being in service to others.

Power Yoga: Ashtanga for Americans

Power yoga is essentially the Americanized interpretation of the Ashtanga-vinyasa yoga method. Yoga teachers Beryl Bender Birch and Bryan Kest coined the term *power yoga* in the late 1980s. Both were practicing Ashtanga-vinyasa yoga at the time, both studied with Sri K. Pattabhi Jois, and both were teaching his method. They agree that they must have come up with the name by simultaneously tapping into the collective unconscious, Birch on the East Coast and Kest on the West Coast. Calling what they were teaching "power yoga" was simply a way of making the fairly esoteric Ashtanga yoga system more accessible to Americans, while letting everyone know that this practice, unlike the majority of yoga taught the 1970s, was a very athletic, intense, sweaty workout designed to build significant strength along with concentration and flexibility. And their tactic worked. The marketing ploy drew hundreds of people through their studio doors and eventually persuaded thousands of Americans to practice yoga. Birch's first book, *Power Yoga* (1995), sold over two hundred thousand copies and was many people's first introduction to yoga. Unfortunately, the name was never trademarked, leaving the style open for interpretation, and pretty soon *everyone* had his or her own version of power yoga: along came power yoga in every gym, as well as Mark Blanchard's Power yoga, Baron Baptiste Power Vinyasa yoga, Reebok Power yoga, and most recently CorePower yoga. Originally closely modeled on the Ashtanga-vinyasa yoga method (even Birch's book *Power Yoga* detailed the system's primary series of poses), power yoga has many different variations today, and the way the style is taught can vary widely from teacher to teacher, depending on who his or her trainer was.

A DIFFERENT KIND OF YOGA

Beryl Bender Birch began practicing yoga in 1971 and had studied Sivananda yoga with Swami Vishnu-devananda, Kundalini yoga with Yogi Bhajan, and Iyengar yoga with senior teachers such as Judith Lasater. Not completely sold on the physical practice just yet, she was instantly captivated with the *rajasic* (active), athletic Ashtanga-vinyasa practice when she attended a workshop led by Norman Allen, Jois's first Western student. His practice was unlike anything she had ever seen before; she immediately began studying with Allen and has been teaching the Ashtanga method or some *vinyasa* variation of the *asana* series since 1980.

In general, power yoga classes are very fitness based and physically demanding. With many of the same elements as an Ashtanga yoga practice — *vinyasa, ujjayi* breath, Sun Salutations, active postures, internal heat, and sweat — power yoga also has many of the same benefits gained from that style of yoga, including increased stamina, strength, balance, and flexibility, as well as detoxification, weight loss, and stress reduction. With both styles rooted in the vigorous *vinyasa* style of Ashtanga yoga, requiring students to synchronize their breath with movement as they flow through a dynamic sequence of postures, variety is the key difference between the two styles. Power yoga does not follow a set series of postures. Teachers creatively design their own class sequences, one pose flowing directly into the next, and their teaching style often develops from their own personal home practice. The presence or absence of any overtly spiritual component is completely dependent on the teacher or the studio, though many would argue it's nearly impossible to take all spirituality out of yoga. That being said, the poses are given in their English names, there usually isn't much chanting or meditation, and any yoga philosophy or wisdom is presented in a very accessible, contextual manner.

THE GOLDEN RULE OF POWER YOGA

The general guiding principle in power yoga is to listen to your body and your breath: If something hurts — stop. If you notice you aren't breathing deeply or can't keep a fullness of breath, back out of the pose. The practice is as much a test of your personal willpower as it is a challenge to surrender when necessary, which isn't an easy feat for those who are used to pushing themselves through their workouts. In class, you are encouraged to skip *vinyasas* or take Child's Pose when it's appropriate for you.

Often billed as a class for athletes, power yoga tends to attract the more fitness-oriented students and sports enthusiasts looking for a strong, balanced workout. However, sometimes the more fit or built you are as an athlete in a particular sport, the more difficult this type of yoga can be, challenging you to access strength and open your body in completely unfamiliar ways. Therefore, no matter how strong or in shape you think you are, you should be cautious about throwing yourself into a power yoga class without first learning the basics from a qualified teacher. Power yoga should be eased into and learned progressively to avoid injury. As in Ashtanga yoga, in power yoga a good teacher will be able to cater to a newcomer. The sort of magic behind the system is that the strong athletic practice attracts people looking to build strength, sweat, and lose weight, but once they're in class, paying attention to their bodies and focusing on their breath, power yoga becomes a work within, and students start to transform from the inside out.

Forrest Yoga: Fierce Medicine

Forrest yoga is an intensely physical practice with a strong internal focus that involves holding poses for extended periods of time in a heated room (usually around 85 degrees). Demanding everything you've got, the vigorous sequences of postures, which emphasize breathing and abdominal work, are designed to build heat and make you sweat, eliminating toxins and releasing emotional and mental tension held in the body. The method, developed by founder Ana Forrest over decades of working through her own healing process, focuses on uncovering unconscious blocks, cleansing and healing deep emotional and psychic pain stored in the cell tissues of our bodies.

Known for her awe-inspiring yoga demonstrations and fierce (sometimes abrasive) teaching style, Ana Forrest has a personal history of abuse, including horrific sexual abuse, epilepsy, bulimia, alcoholism, and drug addiction, which led to the creation of Forrest yoga — a unique combination of physical yoga practices and Eastern and Native American teachings and wisdom. Desperate to alleviate her own pain and suffering, she turned to yoga and just about any healing modality she could find, including various hands-on techniques such as chiropractic, craniosacral, polarity, reflexology, shiatsu, and pressure-point therapy, as well as homeopathic and naturopathic remedies. An ordained practitioner of Native American medicine, a Reiki master, a certified regression therapist, and a graduate of Anthony Robbins Master University, Ana Forrest has spent her lifetime improving herself as a teacher and a gifted healer. In developing and teaching Forrest yoga, she sees herself as doing her part "to mend the hoop of the people — to inspire people to clear through the stuff that hardens them and sickens their bodies so they can walk freely and lightly in a healing way, in a Beauty Way." Her "soul's work" is to teach people how to use the innate wisdom of their bodies to heal themselves and dramatically transform their lives.

A MEDICINAL PRACTICE

On her own quest to heal the afflictions from her battered childhood, Forrest began modifying the yoga postures, creating innovative ways of doing the poses (even new *asanas*) and developing therapeutic sequences to address the chronically "stuck" areas of the body (jaw, neck, shoulders, and hips) as well as other physical ailments that are caused by our modern Western lifestyle. Devoted Forrest yoga students attest that regular practice will alleviate low back pain, relieve chronic tension in the jaw and neck, open hips and shoulders, combat stress, and ease depression.

In her book *Fierce Medicine: Breakthrough Practices to Heal the Body and Ignite the Spirit* (2012), Forrest explains, "Emotions have to be in motion to be healthy. If...they get stashed in the cell tissue...they morph into emotional pus balls. When you're processing a difficult emotional situation, yoga can be powerful medicine." Emotional debris and other junk (such as negative thoughts, experiences, and attitudes) that become trapped in our bodies harden us, eventually making us sick with dis-ease. In Forrest yoga, students are encouraged to turn within and listen to what their bodies are trying to tell them. They learn to become deeply aware of the movement of energy through their bodies, discovering and breathing into the places that are stuck — where emotional pain is lodged, preventing the flow of life force. Forrest yoga is an extremely confrontational method, and there's no escaping or otherwise checking out in class. The best way to describe the practice is the same as the style's founder: fierce. You are forced to dig deep and face whatever emotional, mental, or physical pain or discomfort you've perhaps been able to avoid until now. The practice may not be the most pleasant experience, but it is powerful and indeed therapeutic, evident in the intense sobbing and wails of anger that are common in class.

The method is founded on four pillars: breath, strength, integrity, and spirit. The long, consistent breath awareness taught in Forrest yoga is profound. Students are taught how to feel the breath and to direct and connect it to very specific areas of the body in order to bring not only awareness there but also energy, enlivening every cell in their body. Forrest explains that most of our pain and suffering are the result of unconscious habits or patterns that we fall into, whether they be physical, emotional, mental, or spiritual. For healing to take place, you must break these patterns and establish new ones, beginning with how you breathe. Strength is built through long holds, allowing you to go deeper in the postures, and there is an emphasis on tough abdominal work — your core being your personal center and place of power and strength. Integrity involves knowing how to modify the postures and exercises so that they work best for you and your injuries, emotional as well as physical, while working honestly at your threshold, or edge, where you will begin to develop effective tools for handling stress, fear, and adversities on as well as off your mat.

A strong physical and emotional practice, Forrest yoga aims to deepen your relationship with your authentic Self, your spirit. In her own healing quest, Ana Forrest recognized that along with unconscious patterns and stuck emotions that had hardened her and caused disease, she had lost her spirit. She sought to create a "place in which to welcome your spirit back home." To be clear, she's not teaching transcendence (transcending your body and mind to realize you're nothing other than supreme consciousness) but rather is teaching a strong connection to your deepest truth and authentic gifts, a connection that allows you to live your life according to your intuition, the voice of your spirit. In the end, along with promoting cleaning and healing, the method cultivates personal perseverance, confidence, and the courage to be who you are.

ISHTA Yoga: Science of Self-Transformation

ISHTA yoga integrates the ancient and modern sciences of *hatha*, *tantra*, and ayurveda into one comprehensive system that is designed to help students become more comfortable in themselves, embrace who they are, and create balance in their lives. Asserting that every individual is inherently perfect and that our essential nature is divine and blissful (a distinctly *tantric* belief), the style is a method of self-exploration that offers various tools for discovering and understanding yourself as well as your innate perfection and boundless joy. A completely undogmatic approach, ISHTA yoga caters to the individual, helping students determine which aspects of the vast yoga tradition work best for them and their individual needs — whether that be to gain strength and flexibility, increase vitality, improve mental clarity, create emotional balance, invigorate their life, or deepen their spiritual connection — to find the right combination of yogic practices best suited for their individual paths.

INDIVIDUAL SPIRIT

In addition to serving as an acronym for the "integrated science of *hatha*, *tantra*, and ayurveda," the word *ishta* also appears in Patanjali's Yoga Sutras in a line that translates as "self-study provides the individual with the path to enlightenment." Therefore, *ishta* is taken to mean "individual" and, when expanded, to mean "that which resonates with the individual spirit" in this system of yoga.

Created in South Africa in the late 1960s by Alan Finger and his father, Kavi Yogi Swarananda Mani Finger, ISHTA yoga is a synthesis of their collective studies with many famous gurus and swamis, including Paramahansa Yogananda, the *tantric* master Shuddhand Bharati, Swami Venkatesananda (the "jewel student" of the Sivananda tradition), and Swami Nisreyasananda from the Rama Krishna lineage, as well as B. K. S. Iyengar in his early days. The system continued to be developed, defined, and redefined throughout Alan's teaching career of over forty years, culminating in the opening of the first ISHTA yoga studio on the Upper East Side of Manhattan in 2008 and a second studio opening elsewhere uptown in 2011. Prior to moving to New York, Alan cofounded Yoga Works with Maty Ezraty and Chuck Miller in Los Angeles, then formed the Yoga

Zone studios in New York City in 1993, which became Be Yoga, a hugely successful regional teacher-training program that was incorporated back into the Yoga Works system in 2004. Today ISHTA yoga teachers instruct throughout the United States and Europe as well as in Australia, Canada, Japan, and South Africa.

The modern yoga system is a breath-centered, alignment-oriented practice that combines elements of Ashtanga-vinyasa with the precision of Iyengar yoga and incorporates subtle energy techniques, such as *pranayama* and *kriya* exercises as well as visualization meditations to expand awareness. Revitalizing, strengthening, and aligning the body through sequences of *asanas* and *pranayama*, ISHTA yoga aims to strengthen individual weakness and remove blockages, opening the body's energy channels so that energy can flow freely and bring the body back into balance. Through the practice of *hatha* yoga, students of ISHTA yoga begin to bring their two opposing forces (masculine and feminine, strength and flexibility, hard and soft) into balance. However, *hatha* yoga is just the first step toward uniting the body, mind, and spirit. The physical practice of *asana* and *pranayama* brings the body under control and begins to quiet the mind in preparation for meditation, which is greatly emphasized in ISHTA yoga and considered crucial for personal development and self-transformation.

Integrating the science of *tantra*, the method draws upon *tantric* meditation tools, such as *yantra* forms, *mantra* chants, and visualization techniques, to help students become more aware of the subtler aspects of their beings, harness energy, and elevate their consciousness. While *tantra* is most commonly translated to mean "loom" or "weave," the word is derived from the root verbs *tanoti* (to expand) and *trayati* (to liberate). Grounded in the belief that every individual is part of the divine whole, or the supreme consciousness that pervades everything, *tantra* refers to the expansion of awareness and liberation of individual consciousness in order to experience one's inherent divinity, wholeness, and freedom. And that's just what ISHTA yoga aims to do.

Ayurveda is the system of traditional Indian medicine (dating back at least two thousand years) that focuses on balancing one's personal constitution while considering the individual's lifestyle. According to ayurveda, each of us has his or her own unique constitution, or makeup, which is either positively or negatively affected by the choices we make, whether it be the food we eat, when we sleep, what we practice, how we engage in relationships, or our current situations. Ayurveda (*ayur* meaning "life," and *veda* meaning "knowledge") aims to restore balance on all levels of being and bring the individual back to optimal health and function. In ISHTA yoga, students are encouraged to understand their individual constitutions and to explore how their lifestyles, choices, and circumstances affect their emotional, mental, energetic, and physical well-being. Using the principles of ayurveda, ISHTA yoga teachers help each student address his or her personal imbalances, creating individual physical and spiritual practices just for him or her.

Anusara Yoga: Align with the Divine

Anusara yoga is a very playful approach to *asana* practice aimed at awakening and expressing joy from the inside out. Grounded in the concept of intrinsic goodness — the belief that everyone is free to discover and experience the pure love and delight present within and all around — the school's life-affirming philosophical vision forms the foundation for *asana* practice. Classes tend to be challenging, fun, and upbeat with a clear focus on physical alignment and a heavy injection of spiritual philosophy. Uplifting teachers approach the practice with a can-do attitude, seeking to empower students with a larger sense of personal greatness. In return, Anusara yoga students are expected to be just that, students, there to learn how to safely and optimally align themselves in the poses rather than just "going through" them. The result is a fun-loving community, known as a *kula*, of dedicated (and intelligent) students who embrace the positive and who love exploring new ways of expressing themselves on the mat.

FLOWING WITH GRACE

The word *anusara* means "to be concurrent with grace" (*anu* meaning "concurrent," and *sara* meaning "grace") or "to flow with grace"; the highest intention of Anusara yoga is to "align with the Divine," meaning to align with your true nature and awaken to the inherent goodness eternally present in yourself and others. By stepping deeper into the currents of grace, moving into alignment with your own heart, you become more and more yourself.

The school of Anusara yoga was founded and created by John Friend. Originally an Iyengar yoga teacher (certified at the junior intermediate level), Friend was profoundly influenced by the spiritual leader Gurumayi Chidvilasananda, head of the Siddha yoga lineage. He was captivated by her teachings and *tantric* philosophy, and ideas of nondualism and the transcendence of grace began to creep into his teaching. Furthermore, having studied biomechanics and kinesiology during his years in the Iyengar system, he began to develop and teach his own way of organizing the alignment principles, straying away from the traditional Iyengar method. Feeling that he was no longer honoring the Iyengar method, which is founded on a dual classical yoga philosophy, Friend resigned and set out to create his own system of yoga, combining alignment principles with a nondual *tantric* philosophy, and in 1997 Friend birthed Anusara yoga.

Named as one of "the World's Greatest Yoga Masters" in the June 2007 issue of *Vanity Fair*, Friend was one of the most sought-after yoga teachers worldwide until February 2012, when a large scandal broke, forcing the founder to resign after much deliberation. Once one of the fastest-growing schools in the world, Anusara yoga took a large hit, losing hundreds, if not thousands, of teachers who no longer list their classes under the trademarked Anusara name. Reforming as a teacher-led organization, the Anusara School of Hatha Yoga emerged and, according to the school's website, continues to uphold the high standards of Anusara yoga created by Friend, including the extremely rigorous teacher certification process he designed, and hopes to rebuild the powerhouse that Anusara yoga once was. (For a current listing of certified Anusara yoga teachers, please visit the Anusara School of Hatha Yoga's website.)

After years of studying and teaching yoga (primarily Iyengar, which he taught for over a decade), Friend began to realize that each teacher gave his or her own instructions on a variety of points to achieve optimal alignment in different postures. Thinking it would be easier for students if the alignment instructions could be organized into succinct principles, Friend studied the biomechanics of over 250 poses and found a very distinct pattern. That pattern became Anusara yoga's trademarked Universal Principles of Alignment (UPAs). Applied in the same order in every single *asana*, the UPAs consist of five common steps that work in balance to bring the body into physical alignment by breaking down the technical instructions into easily understood elements.

UNIVERSAL PRINCIPLES OF ALIGNMENT

OPEN TO GRACE: Expanding the inner body, softening the outer boundaries, setting the foundation and intention

MUSCULAR ENERGY: Hugging the muscles to the bone, hugging to the midline, and drawing in from the periphery to the focal point

INNER SPIRAL: Internally rotating the legs, thighs, and pelvis

OUTER SPIRAL: Externally rotating the legs, thighs, and pelvis

ORGANIC ENERGY: Expanding from bones to skin, extending from the focal point in all directions

The belief that we are all divine consciousness permeates every aspect of Anusara yoga. The two main purposes for practicing are to remember that you are nothing but divinity, realizing your innate power and beauty, and to celebrate your embodiment of divine consciousness. Every class begins with the delivery of a philosophical, or "heart-oriented," theme (typically centered on cultivating a virtuous quality, such as courage or compassion). The opening theme is meant to give you an attitudinal direction, or an intention, for your *asana* practice. Sharing relevant personal stories, imparting teachings from sacred texts, and illustrating with analogies and metaphors, the teacher will continue to carry the theme throughout class, interweaving the style's life-affirming *tantric* philosophy with technical alignment instructions — seeking to infuse the physical practice with meaning.

Classes in general are appropriate for a range of ages and ability levels. Trained to assess the room for ability and attitude and to structure the class accordingly, Anusara yoga teachers will modify postures with props when necessary or offer advanced variations of poses for students ready to attempt the next level of *asana*. More or fewer alignment instructions are given depending on the level of the class, assuming that if you're attending a more advanced class you have a clear understanding of the UPAs, and teachers will always offer individual feedback, actively making verbal and manual adjustments when necessary. As a whole the system loves handstands and doesn't hold back from inversions and arm balances, and partner work may or may not be involved. Most Anusara yoga classes also have a strong emphasis on heart-opening poses (backbends). However, in the end, the overriding purpose of class is for the student to feel better when leaving than when he or she walked in, emotionally, spiritually, and physically.

Moksha Yoga: Freedom to Be You

A fast-growing form of hot yoga, Moksha yoga is a well-balanced series of forty postures that begins and ends with Savasana. The style was founded in Toronto in 2004 by experienced yoga teachers Ted Grand and Jessica Robertson after the partners realized that what they were offering in their Canadian Bikram yoga studios wasn't in line with Bikram's strict guidelines. For starters, their studios weren't carpeted, they were using props and modifying the postures (a huge no-no in Bikram yoga), and they weren't teaching from the scripted Bikram dialogue. Quite to the contrary, although all Moksha yoga classes are rooted in the Bikram style's set series, Moksha yoga teachers (many of whom have studied multiple yoga systems) are encouraged to incorporate their individual knowledge and expertise, drawing from their own experiences and personal practices. Teachers are even invited to set an intention, or theme, for their class, and often most do, bringing different elements of the hot yoga practice into focus and showcasing their creativity.

Other discrepancies from Bikram yoga include Moksha yoga's focus on building upper-body strength (the Moksha series does in fact incorporate Down Dog), as well as the *asana* series' emphasis on opening the hips, which helps prevent and alleviate lower back and knee pain. To help you relax and let go of any expectations you may be placing on yourself or your practice or both, class begins with lying flat on your back in Savasana, allowing your central nervous system to decompress before the challenging cardiovascular practice. Once class is under way, students work through the standing series of postures, holding each for anywhere from ten to sixty seconds, allowing the body to build heat and sweat out toxins. Then it's on to the floor series of postures that work on strengthening the upper body, spine, and abdominal core muscles, as well as opening the hips now that the body is warm. Class ends where it began, in Savasana, after which students leave at their own pace, feeling lighter, happier, and a bit shinier. Moksha yoga shares many of the same benefits of any hot yoga practice, including cardiovascular health, detoxification, stress reduction, weight loss, increased metabolism, relief from depression, and better sleep rhythms.

ONE SERIES, MULTIPLE CLASSES

Traditionally, the Moksha yoga series of forty postures is completed in a ninety-minute practice; however, studios also offer a condensed version of the series in sixty- and seventy-five-minute classes. Other variations on the same series include Moksha flow, which adds *vinyasas* between the postures; practice to Moksha music, in which the series is executed to a great playlist; and silent Moksha, during which the class is led by the breath and by the teacher practicing on his or her mat.

What began with the vision of two individuals has grown into a worldwide sweaty Moksha yoga community, with over thirty affiliated studios in Canada, the United States, Switzerland, and the Caribbean. Each studio is independently owned by a certified yoga teacher and approved by the style's founders. At the heart of all Moksha yoga studios are the style's seven pillars: be healthy, be accessible, live green, participate in *sangha* (or community) support, reach out, live to learn, and be at peace. Every associated studio must adhere to fairly strict "green" standards, including the use of sustainable building materials and natural cleaning products, and remain committed to leading environmentally conscious lives. According to the belief that yoga should be made accessible to all, anyone and everyone is welcome in Moksha yoga; teachers truly want you to feel at home in their studios, whether you're a corporate CEO or a peace crusader. The teachers use common and clear language throughout class and, as mentioned before, offer props and modifications. So you don't have to be flexible to come to class; just come as you are, and the teacher will help you access the poses.

Ultimately, Moksha yoga is all about community, specifically about a community of teachers and students supporting one another on their own individual paths of growth and positive change. Moksha yoga teachers strive to create a place where everyone feels as if he or she belongs and is part of something special. In 2007, Moksha yoga helped form the New Leaf Yoga Foundation, which brings free yoga programs to high-risk and incarcerated youth. In addition to that, all studios offer by-donation, or *karma*, classes at least once a week, with the proceeds being donated to local charities and environmental efforts. Through Moksha yoga's dedicated studio owners, teachers, and students, the community — or family, as they so lovingly refer to themselves — is flourishing and continues to evolve as the style builds more of a presence in the yoga community at large.

FREEDOM

Moksha means "freedom or liberation." The most literal Indian definition of *moksha* is "freedom, or liberation, from the cycles of birth and death." Moksha yoga is the invitation to discover what freedom means to you personally, whether it's freedom from chronic tension or pain in the body, freedom from self-judgment or criticism, or simply an hour and a half of freedom from the demands of your hectic life.

AcroYoga: Playful Partner Practice

AcroYoga is a partner-based practice that blends the teachings and wisdom of yoga with the power and playfulness of acrobatics and the sensitivity and loving touch of healing arts. Partners work together to create new openings in the body while exploring aerial movements and postures in a safe, accepting atmosphere, with one partner acting as the base and the second as the flier. Most often, the base lies flat on his or her back with legs extended straight up, aligning the ankles over the hips and stacking the bones of the legs to support the flier on his or her feet. Once properly stacked, the legs can actually support a considerable amount of weight, allowing a smaller person to safely fly a bigger partner. The person in the air can be supported in a number of ways, the most basic being by the hips for superman-style flying, passive forward folds, or backbends. Oftentimes a third person will act as a spotter, serving as the intermediary between the base and the flier and aiding in the stability of the flight by making sure everyone maintains good alignment to prevent the flier from falling. Once the flier is back on the ground, he or she gives the base partner a Thai yoga massage as a thank-you for the flight.

THE MAGIC WORD

Clear communication is a crucial component of AcroYoga, in the cultivation of listening, sensitivity, and trust. *Down* is the magic word. At any time, if the flier or the base partner feels uncomfortable, he or she just says "down," and the flier is let down safely.

Relatively new on the yoga scene, AcroYoga was cofounded by Jason Nemer and Jenny Saver, who began practicing together in 2002. Combining their collective backgrounds in aerobics, circus arts, and yoga, they began to explore and create supported aerial versions of the classic yoga postures. The cofounders went on to develop a progressive, systematic approach that involves two forms of flying: acrobatic and therapeutic, making the practice accessible to just about everyone. Their intention was always to cultivate connection, community, and trust through direct interaction. AcroYoga was officially labeled in 2006 and has been gaining popularity ever since. Nemer attributes the style's rapid growth to its ability to bring people together in support of one another for the purpose of play, especially in a world that has become increasingly cyber-oriented.

Every AcroYoga class begins with an opening circle, during which all participants introduce themselves and share a little bit about what's going on in their bodies, specifically any injuries or limitations. The opening circle also sets the intention for class, whether the focus will be acrobatic or therapeutic. Basically an inverted aerial massage, therapeutic flying involves sensitivity, mindfulness, loving touch, and letting go — using gravity to gently release and open the flier's spine with a supported inversion. The flier, supported by the base's legs, hangs passively while the base partner uses his or her hands to lightly stretch and massage the flier's upper body. Once down, the flier then massages the base's legs, which are nice and warm. The session is over when both partners have flown and based and have had the opportunity to both give and receive (a fundamental concept of AcroYoga). On the other hand, acrobatic flying is dynamic; both the base and the flier are active participants in creating an aerial flow from pose to pose, requiring cooperation and trust. The creative opportunities to join their bodies in supported flight are endless; the practice itself, playful and empowering. Acroyogis are known for their impromptu "jam" outdoor sessions, during which partners play around for fun, exploring new movements and poses. Acrobatic flying involves a showmanship that is graceful.

THREE MAIN ELEMENTS

AcroYoga has three main elements: solar acrobatic, lunar therapeutic, and yogic practices. Solar acrobatic practices involve building strength, particularly core strength, inversions, and partner acrobatics. Lunar therapeutic practices involve massage techniques and therapeutic flying. And the yogic practices and life philosophies are the foundation for both solar and lunar practices, cultivating breath awareness, self-reflection, and connection.

CONCLUSION

Now that you've read about various yoga styles and are more familiar with the different approaches to practicing, hopefully you've found a system of yoga that resonates with you. Even if you're still unsure about certain elements of a style's practice, try a class anyway — you may surprise yourself. Sometimes we need to nudge ourselves out of our comfort zones in order to discover things about ourselves we may not otherwise come to know. You'll find that most yoga teachers create a very safe and supportive environment for you to try new things, expand your boundaries, and let your guard down a bit. Attend weekly classes and you'll quickly find yourself a part of a community — a yoga tribe, so to speak. You may never see your fellow students outside of the yoga studio, but within the confines of class you'll share challenges and struggles as well as breakthroughs and triumphs. You'll try things with your body that you would be hesitant to do in front of your spouse or best friend. A certain level of intimacy is created, so be aware of that as you begin to immerse yourself in a yoga style and community, and choose accordingly.

At some point in time, you may also discover that you're bored with your yoga practice, or that your needs or interests have changed. Or perhaps a teacher whom you love is moving away, presenting you with the opportunity to discover what else is out there in terms of yoga practice. When the time is right, revisit *Pick Your Yoga Practice* and you may notice that you're now interested in offerings and practices that weren't for you the first time around.

Also, be aware that you may fall out of practice from time to time; most of us do, and that's okay. Yoga isn't going anywhere. When you're ready, you'll make your way back to your mat. Sometimes you must forget for a while in order to remember why you fell in love with the practice in the beginning. Yoga isn't about getting anywhere or proving anything. It's about growing as an individual, becoming more yourself, finding more clarity and ease in your life, and living more fully. So don't beat yourself up. Just unroll your mat and start practicing again. Your body will remember, and your teacher and classmates will welcome you back, no questions asked.

The most important thing to remember is that this is your yoga practice, your time on your mat with your body and breath. If something doesn't feel right, or hurts (as opposed to just being uncomfortable or challenging), don't do it. Don't be disrespectful to the teacher, but always respect your body's needs and limitations, as well as your personal boundaries. Conversely, don't become too caught up in pleasing the teacher or impressing your fellow classmates. Push yourself to work hard, rest when you need to, and modify the practice as necessary. If there comes a time and place in which you don't feel respected or feel violated in any way, then it's most likely time to find a new teacher, or even to search for a new system whose philosophy and values are more in line with your own. Again, return to this book. You'll most likely have a new perspective now that you've been around the yoga block a few times.

As a yoga teacher and someone who doesn't know what she'd do or where she'd be without her yoga practice, I'm thrilled you've found your way to *Pick Your Yoga Practice*. I truly hope that you find the yoga style, teacher, and community that uplift and fulfill you, support and heal you, and comfort and guide you as you journey deeper into your own heart.

Namaste.

ACKNOWLEDGMENTS

First, I'd like to express my gratitude for all the teachers who have influenced my yogic path, as well as my students, without whom I wouldn't get to do what I love most — teach yoga. Second, I'd like to thank all of the leading yoga teachers who were so generous with their time and willingness to be interviewed for this book: Swami Asokananda, Beryl Bender Birch, Ana Brett and Ravi Singh, Rajashree Choudhury, Nischala Joy Devi, Sandhi Ferreira, Naime Jezzeny, Sudha Carolyn Lundeen, Noah Mazé, Elise Browning Miller, Kia Miller, Tim Miller, Swami Ramananda, Desiree Rumbaugh, John Schumacher, and Joan White.

A great big thanks to my agent, Elizabeth Evans, who encouraged me to put this book out there and was a huge support throughout the entire process, advocating on my behalf and rooting me on to the end. I also thank my editors, Georgia Hughes and Kristen Cashman, for being so supportive, gracious, and good at what they do, along with my publicist, Kim Corbin, and the rest of the staff at New World Library.

I'd also like to thank my thesis adviser, Madelyn Cain-Inglese; without her encouragement I would have given up on writing altogether.

I am eternally grateful to my parents, family, and friends, who not only knew I could do it and cheered me on but also allowed me to fall apart when the stress got the better of me. And a special thanks to James Ford for living through this process with me; I know it wasn't always easy.

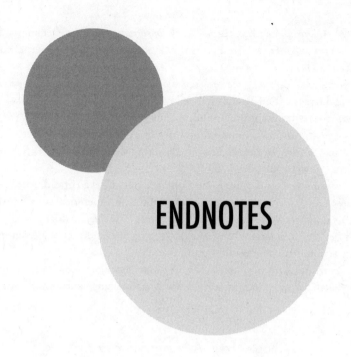

ENDNOTES

Introduction

Page xi *"the 'virtuosity in becoming yourself'"*: Chris Calarco, "Class Theme and Contemplations Week of 5/8/13," *Chris Calarco Yoga* (blog), July 1, 2013, chriscalarco yoga.com/2013/05/class-themes-and-contemplations-week-of-may-6-2013/.

Chapter One. Yoga Explained

Page 16 *"In the beginner's mind there are many possibilities..."*: Mary Jaksch, "How to Live Life to the Max with Beginner's Mind," *Zen Habits* (blog), July 1, 2013, zenhabits.net/how-to-live-life-to-the-max-with-beginners-mind.

Chapter Two. America's Yoga History

Page 22 *"Yoga is the cessation of the fluctuations of the mind"*: Ann Pizer, "Yoga Chitta Vritti Nirodha," About.com, May 22, 2013, Yoga.about.com/od/yogaquotes/qt /Yoga-Chitta-Vritti-Nirodha.htm.
Page 24 *"are but various phases of one eternal religion"*: Pravrajika Vrajaprana, "A Vedanta Way of Life," Vedanta Society of Southern California, May 22, 2013, vedanta.org/2001/monthly-readings/a-vedanta-way-of-life.

Page 25 *"In America is the place, the people, the opportunity…"*: Holly Hammond, "Yoga's Trip to America," *Yoga Journal*, May 22, 2013, www.yogajournal.com /wisdom/467.

Page 25 *"to disseminate among the nations a knowledge…"*: Paramahansa Yogananda, "Aims and Ideals of Self-Realization Fellowship," Self-Realization Fellowship, May 22, 2013, www.yogananda-srf.org/Aims_and_Ideals.aspx#.UZ6VqGQ5yK8.

Page 29 *"yoga to be India's greatest gift to the world"*: R. H. Cravens and T. K. V. Desikachar, *Health, Healing & Beyond: Yoga and the Living Tradition of T. Krishnamacharya* (New York: North Point Press, 2011), 123.

Page 30 *"woman who brought yoga to the Kremlin"*: Meta Chaya Hirschl, *Vital Yoga: A Sourcebook for Students and Teachers* (New York: The Experiment, LLC, 2011), 42.

Page 31 *"immediately fell in love with the country and its people"*: Adriana Aboy, "Indra Devi's Legacy," *Hinduism Today*, May 22, 2013, www.hinduismtoday.com/modules /smartsection/item.php?itemid=3846.

Page 33 *"America is becoming a whole…"*: Sri Swami Satchidananda, "Woodstock," Sri Swami Satchidananda, May 25, 2013, www.swamisatchidananda.org/docs2/wood stock.htm.

Chapter Four. Ashtanga-vinyasa Yoga

Page 49 *"If we practice the science of yoga…"*: Waylon Lewis, "Pattabhi Jois, Founder of Ashtanga Yoga, Passes Away at Age 93," *Huffington Post*, May 9, 2013, www .huffingtonpost.com/waylon-lewis/pattabhi-jois-founder-of_b_204938.html.

Page 50 *"Ashtanga yoga method is Patanjali Yoga"*: "Ashtanga's Eight Limbs of Yoga," *About-Yoga*, May 9, 2013, www.about-yoga.com/ashtanga-eight-limbs.html.

Page 57 *Ashtanga yoga opening and closing chants*: "Yoga Chants," Ashtanga Workshop, May 7, 2013, www.ashtangaworkshop.com/ashtanga_chants.php.

Page 60 *"Do not do yoga without* vinyasa*"*: "Traditional and Guided Classes," Shri K. Pattabhi Jois Ashtanga Yoga Institute, May 9, 2013, kpjayi.org/the-practice /traditional-method.

Page 61 *"Without* bandhas, *breathing will not be correct…"*: "The Practice," Shri K. Pattabhi Jois Ashtanga Yoga Institute, July 9, 2013, kpjayi.org/the-practice.

Chapter Five. Iyengar Yoga

Page 65 *"Health is a state of complete harmony of the body…"*: Jason Wachob, "B. K. S. Iyengar Turns 92 Today: Yoga and Your Health," *Mind Body Green*, May 9, 2013, www.mindbodygreen.com/0-1770/BKS-Iyengar-Turns-92-Today-Yoga-and -Your-Health.html.

Page 71 *Invocation to Sage Patanjali*: "Invocation to Sage Patanjali by Iyengar," B. K. S. Iyengar Yoga, May 7, 2013, www.bksiyengar.com/modules/IYoga /sage.htm.

Chapter Six. Kundalini Yoga

Page 81 *"Kundalini yoga classes are a dynamic blend…"*: Yogi Bhajan, "About Kundalini Yoga," Kundalini Yoga Center, May 8, 2013, www.kundaliniyogacenter .com/aboutyoga.htm.

Page 101 "ong namo guru dev namo": *"Mantras,"* Kundalini Yoga, May 8, 2013, www.kundaliniyoga.org/*mantra*.html.

Chapter Seven. Integral Yoga

Page 105 *"Integral Yoga is a flexible combination…"*: "What Is Integral Yoga," Integral Yoga Institute San Francisco, May 9, 2013, www.integralyogasf.org/about.html.

Page 106 *"The entire world is going to watch this.…"*: "The History of Integral Yoga," Integral Yoga Institute New York City, May 9, 2013, www.iyiny.org/about/the _history_of_integral_yoga.

Page 114 *"The goal of Integral yoga…"*: His Holiness Sri Swami Satchidananda, "The Goal of Integral Yoga," Integral Yoga Institute New York City, May 9, 2013, www.iyiny.org/about/the_goal_of_integral_yoga.

Page 117 "karma *yoga alone is enough to save your soul."*: Sri Swami Satchidananda, "The Greatness of Karma Yoga," Yogaville Satchidananda Ashram, May 9, 2013, www.yogaville.org/2012/02/the-greatness-of-karma-yoga.

Chapter Eight. Kripalu Yoga

Page 121 *"Kripalu is the first traditional yoga* ashram *founded…"*: "History," Kripalu, May 8, 2013, www.kripalu.org/about_us/5.

Page 136 *"journey from the known to the unknown"*: Richard Faulds, "The Journey from Known to Unknown," Kripalu, July 12, 2013, www.kripalu.org/kyta_artcl.l.php ?id=177.

Chapter Nine. Bikram Yoga

Page 139 *"Your mind is your number one enemy.…"*: Jocasta Shakespeare, "Bend It Like Bikram," *The Observer*, June 10, 2006, www.guardian.co.uk/lifeandstyle/2006/jun /11/healthandwellbeing.features1.

Page 140 *"energized from the inside out"*: Debra Carr-Elsing, "Taking Flexibility to the Max," *Capital Times*, January 2, 2003, www.bikramyoga.com/News/press17.php.

Chapter Ten. Jivamukti Yoga

Page 153 *"Jivamukti yoga incorporates traditional yoga practices…"*: Sharon Gannon and David Life, *Jivamukti Yoga: Practices for Liberating Body and Soul* (New York: Ballantine Publishing Company, 2002), 7–8.

Page 155 *"May all living beings, everywhere, ..."*: Gannon and Life, *Jivamukti Yoga*, 78.

Page 156 *"You are not the body and mind..."*: Gannon and Life, *Jivamukti Yoga*, 86.

Page 157 *"making yoga cool and hip"*: "Spiritual Stretching: The Yoga Portfolio," *Vanity Fair*, June 2007.

Page 163 *"based on the old paradigm..."*: Catherine Clyne, "Jivamukti: Teaching Peace," *Satya Magazine*, June 2006, accessed on Jivamukti Yoga website, May 10, 2013, jivamuktiyoga.com/teachings/published-articles/p/jivamukti-teaching -peace.

Page 163 *"What could be more physical than what we eat, ..."*: "Activism," Jivamukti Yoga, May 10, 2013, www.jivamuktiyoga.com/about/activism.

Page 165 *"no point in practicing asanas"*: Rachel Flax, "Respectable Re-presentation or 'Exotic Chic' Consumerism: A Case Study of the Trendiest Yoga Center in New York City," Hinduism Here: Barnard College and Columbia University, July 12, 2003, barnard.edu/hinduismhere/rachel.html.

Chapter Eleven. Best of the Rest

Page 168 *"future leaders and responsible citizens of the world..."*: "True World Order," International Sivananda Yoga Vedanta Centers, May 9, 2013, www.sivananda.org /about/two.html.

Page 171 *"drawing the cosmic energy into the body..."*: "The Energization Exercises of Paramhansa Yogananda," Ananda Sangha, May 9, 2013, www.ananda.org /meditation/free-meditation-support/meditation-techniques/the-energization -exercises-of-paramhansa-yogananda/.

Page 171 *"portal through which the energy enters the body"* and *"the mouth of God"*: "The Energization Exercises of Paramhansa Yogananda," Ananda Sangha Worldwide, July 13, 2003, www.ananda.org/meditation/free-meditation-support/meditation -techniques/the-energization-exercises-of-paramhansa-yogananda/.

Page 174 *"the bliss of your own being"*: "Discover an Innovative Approach to an Ancient Practice," Svaroopa Yoga, July 13, 2013, www.svaroopayoga.org.

Page 175 *"to know yourself at the deepest level..."*: Judith Lasater, "Definition and Heart of Yoga," Judith Hanson Lasater, PhD, PT, May 25, 2013, www.judithlasater .com/writings/tensutras.html.

Page 176 *"all a function of grace"*: "Founding Master Yoga," Master Yoga Foundation, July 15, 2013, www.svaroopayoga.org/swamiji.html.

Page 176 *"He gave it to me in one instant..."*: "Origin of Svaroopa Yoga," Master Yoga Foundation, July 15, 2013, www.svaroopayoga.org/swamiji.html.

Page 180 *"to mend the hoop of the people..."*: "About Ana T. Forrest," Forrest Yoga, May 9, 2013, www.forrestyoga.com/about.

Page 180 *"Emotions have to be in motion..."*: Jamie Stringfellow, "Embodying Change: How Movement Can Transform Your Life," Spirituality and Health, July 15, 2013,

Spiritualityhealth.com/articles/embodying-change-how-movement-can
-transform-your-life#sthash.LUf1f39y.dpuf.

Page 181 *"place in which to welcome your spirit back home"*: "Forrest Yoga Philosophy,"
Forrest Yoga, May 2013, www.forrestyoga.com/about/philosophy.php.

Page 182 *"self-study provides the individual with..."*: Ishtayogaeurope.com/ishtayoga
/blog/1002, April 6, 2013.

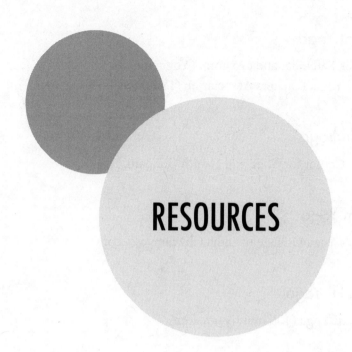

RESOURCES

Ashtanga-vinyasa Yoga

Shri K. Pattabhi Jois Ashtanga Yoga Institute (KPJAYI.org)
Ashtanga Yoga Center (Ashtangayogacenter.com)

Iyengar Yoga

Iyengar Yoga, National Association of the United States (IYNAUS.org)
Ramamani Iyengar Memorial Yoga Institute (BKSIyengar.com)

Kundalini Yoga

Healthy, Happy, Holy Organization (3HO.org)
International Kundalini Teachers Association (IKYT.org)

Integral Yoga

Yogaville Satchidananda Ashram (Yogaville.org)
Integral Yoga Teachers Association (IYTA.org)

Kripalu Yoga

Kripalu Center for Yoga and Health (Kripalu.org)

Bikram Yoga

Bikram's Yoga College of India (Bikramyoga.com)

Jivamukti Yoga

Jivamukti Yoga (Jivamuktiyoga.com)

Sivananda Yoga

International Sivananda Yoga Vedanta Centers (Sivananda.org)

Ananda Yoga

Ananda Sangha Worldwide (Ananda.org)

Viniyoga

American Viniyoga Institute (Viniyoga.com)

Svaroopa Yoga

Master Yoga Foundation (Svaroopayoga.org)

Power Yoga

Bryan Kest's Power Yoga (Poweryoga.com)
The Hard & The Soft Yoga Institute (power-yoga.com)

Forrest Yoga

Forrest Yoga (Forrestyoga.com)

ISHTA Yoga

Ishta Yoga (Ishtayoga.com)

Anusara Yoga

Anusara School of Hatha Yoga (Anusarayoga.com)

Moksha Yoga

Moksha Yoga International (Mokshayoga.ca)

AcroYoga

AcroYoga (Acroyoga.org)

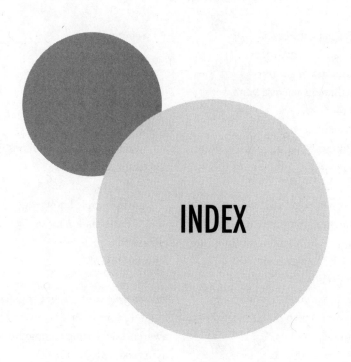

INDEX

ABOUT THE AUTHOR

Meagan McCrary is a certified yoga instructor and freelance writer. Her teaching path has been greatly influenced by Anusara yoga founder John Friend as well as Noah Mazé, Elena Brower, and Martin and Jordan Kirk. Her yoga, wellness, and lifestyle writings are widely featured in print and online in publications including *Elephant Journal*, *GaiamLife*, and *Glo*. She is also coauthor, with Natasha Burton and Julie Fishman, of *The Little Black Book of Big Red Flags: Relationship Warning Signs You Totally Spotted but Chose to Ignore*. She lives in Los Angeles, California, where she teaches at various Equinox Sports Clubs, and offers yoga retreats nationally and internationally. Visit her online at www.MeaganMcCrary.com.